UROLOGY
AND
REPRODUCTION

The REGENTS/PRENTICE HALL
MEDICAL ASSISTANT KIT

UROLOGY AND REPRODUCTION

Third Edition

REGENTS/PRENTICE HALL, Englewood Cliffs, New Jersey 07632

Library of Congress Cataloging in Publication Data

Urology and reproduction. — 3rd. ed.
        p. cm. — (The Regents/Prentice Hall medical assistant kit)
    Rev. ed. of Urology and the male reproductive system / [by
Elizabeth K. White]. 2nd ed. c1984.
    Includes index.
    ISBN 0-13-035676-X
    1. Urinary organs—Diseases. 2. Urology. 3. Generative organs-
-Diseases. 4. Human reproduction. 5. Medical assistants.
I. White, Elizabeth K.   Urology and the male reproductive system.
II. Regents/Prentice Hall.   III. Title: Urology and reproduction.
IV. Series.
    [DNLM: 1. Reproduction. 2. Urology.   WJ 100 U7931]
    RC871.W58 1992
    616.6—dc20
    DNLM/DLC
    for Library of Congress   92-48863
                                                              CIP

© 1993 by REGENTS/PRENTICE HALL
A division of Simon & Schuster
Englewood Cliffs, NJ 07632

Notice

The information and procedures described in the REGENTS/PRENTICE HALL MEDICAL
ASSISTANT KIT are based on consultation with practitioners and instructors and are to be
used as part of a formal course taught by a qualified Medical Assistant instructor. To the best of
the publisher's knowledge, this information reflects currently accepted practices; however, it
cannot be considered absolute recommendations. For individual application, the policies and
procedures of the institution or agency where the Medical Assistant is employed must be
reviewed and followed. The authors of these materials and their supplements disclaim
responsiblity for any adverse effects resulting directly or indirectly from the suggested procedures and theory, from any undetected errors, or from the reader's misunderstanding of the
materials. It is the reader's responsiblity to stay informed of any new changes or recommendations made by his or her employing health care institution or agency.

Printed in the United States of America

10   9   8   7   6   5   4   3   2   1

ISBN   0-13-035676-X

Prentice-Hall International (UK) Limited, *London*
Prentice-Hall of Australia, Pty Limited, *Sydney*
Prentice-Hall Canada, Inc., *Toronto*
Prentice-Hall Hispanoamericana, S.A., *Mexico*
Prentice-Hall of India Private Limited, *New Delhi*
Prentice-Hall of Japan, Inc., *Tokyo*
Simon & Schuster Asia Pte. Ltd., *Singapore*
Editora Prentice-Hall do Brasil, Ltda., *Rio de Janeiro*

Contents

Preface

The REGENTS/PRENTICE HALL MEDICAL ASSISTANT KIT is the only textbook series written for students of Medical Assisting, which integrates the study of anatomy and physiology with diagnosis and treatment of disease. Our goal in this revision was to update and improve the series.

To achieve this goal, we solicited the advice of long-time users of the kit. Their comments resulted in many basic changes including simplification of concepts and procedures; addition of up-to-date information; an emphasis on quality control in all aspects of the physician's office laboratory; and enhanced study aids.

SIMPLIFICATION AND UP-TO-DATE INFORMATION

- All the books are infection-control–conscious throughout, reflecting the latest OSHA regulations.
- Anatomy and physiology titles have been simplified to reflect the very practical approach taken by many instructors.
- Diagnoses and treatments of disease have been up-dated for each body system.
- A thoroughly revised *Bio-Organization* launches the anatomy and physiology series with a simplified introduction to the structure and function of the body and a solid foundation for the study of human disease.
- *Laboratory Processes for Medical Assisting* is revised with more than 60 percent new material including performance-based procedure checklists for easy instructor evaluation, and the latest requirements of the Clinical Laboratory Improvement Act (CLIA).
- *Clinical Processes for Medical Assisting* now emphasizes only clinical procedures in the POL, leaving administrative issues to other more specific courses.

EMPHASIS ON QUALITY CONTROL

As the federal, state and local regulations become more specific, it is clear that the physician's major challenge is to provide not only the highest level of quality care and treatment for the patient, but also to document his or her commitment to that quality for the interest of government. It most often falls on the shoulders of the medical assistant to execute and police the quality control procedures within the office. The new laboratory books emphasize this need for quality control documentation.

The popular "Sources of Error" within the laboratory and clinical procedures checklists have been scrutinized and amplified.

ENHANCED STUDY AIDS

- Knowledge Objectives are grouped by chapter and by section.
- Pronunciations of medical terms are provided the first time a word is used. New terms appear in bold type and are defined in the extensive updated glossary.
- STOP AND REVIEW sections reflect Knowledge Objectives by section or by chapter.
- Over 60 new or revised illustrations and tables complement the text.
- All illustrations and tables are now precisely referenced in the text.
- Contemporary "sidebars" add spice and topical information to entice the student.
- Redesigned books emphasize organization and easy reading.
- Two new simplified four-color inserts are: A blood cell chart showing normal and abnormal blood cells; and 12 pages of body systems illustrations to accompany the *Bio-Organization* introduction.
- *Clinical Processes for Medical Assisting* includes the same type procedure checklist as *Laboratory Processes for Medical Assisting* for easy instructor evaluation.
- The laboratory books contain both Knowledge Objectives and Terminal Performance Objectives.

PREVIOUS BENEFITS RETAINED

The same strengths and benefits which instructors valued in the past have been retained or expanded:

- The flexible modular format can adjust to various program lengths or different orders of coverage for laboratory, clinical, and anatomy and physiology topics.
- The kit is written in a style specifically appropriate to the medical assisting student.
- The text/workbook style aids student learning. The material remains in small, manageable segments.
- The kit takes an integrated approach to structure, function, and disease of the human body.
- Each body system or medical specialty is followed by its clinical counterpoint of disease, diagnosis and treatment.
- A thorough review of disorders and diseases is classified by type in *Bio-Organization*, and by system through the subsequent anatomy and physiology 10-book series.
- The kit features an emphasis on quality control in *Laboratory Processes for Medical Assisting* and *Clinical Processes for Medical Assisting*.
- No prior knowledge of biology or chemistry is assumed.

ACKNOWLEDGMENTS

The revision of the Medical Assistant Kit represents a cooperative effort among many people. Foremost is Debra Grieneisen, M.T., C.M.A., who served as advisor for the series and in-depth reviser for *Laboratory Process for Medical Assisting*. Debra has taught medical assisting at Harrisburg Area Community College and Central Pennsylvania Business School, and it is her commitment to perfection that guided this work.

Several medical writers contributed to these books. Thank you to:

Karen Garloff, R.N.
Bruce Goldfarb
Steve Hulse
Ann Moy
Joy Nixon, R.N.

Cindy Jennings of BMR led the editorial efforts to manage this revision. Helping her were Nancy Priff and Rick Stull, as well as Jacqueline Flynn and Greg Flynn.

We particularly want to thank the reviewers whose advice, recommendations and collective knowledge helped form these books. Their concern for the subject matter, its accuracy, and primarily their students' best interest are reflected here. One thing they all agreed upon is the importance of accurate, clear illustrations which are integrated and referenced throughout the text. Our reviewers were:

Joanne Bakel
    Milton S. Hershey Medical
    Center
    Hershey, PA

Linda Barrer
    Lansdale Business School
    Lansdale, PA

Judy Bettinger
    Private Medical Practice
    Camp Hill, PA

C. Michael Cronin
    California College of Health
    Sciences
    National City, CA

Martha Faison
    Private Medical Practice
    Camp Hill, PA

Irene Figliolina
    Berdan Institute
    Totowa, NJ

Kathleen Hess
    Antonelli Medical &
    Professional Institute
    Pottstown, PA

Carol Kish
    Harrisburg Hospital
    Harrisburg, PA

Peter Kish
    Harrisburg Area Community
    College
    Harrisburg, PA

Tibby Loveman
    Gadsden Business College
    Gadsden, AL

Scott McKenzie
    Commonwealth College
    Virginia Beach, VA

Pat Morelli
    Medical Careers Training
    Center
    Ft. Collins, CO

Rhonda O'Grady
    The Laboratory Arts Institute
    Scarborough, Ontario

Sheila Ritchey
    Harrisburg Hospital
    Harrisburg, PA

Sandy Rishell
    Private Medical Practice
    Harrisburg, PA
Janet Sesser
    The Bryman School
    Phoenix, AZ
Shirley Seekford
    Antonelli Medical &
    Professional Institute
    Pottstown, PA
Robert Sheperd Kee
    Business College
    Norfolk, VA
Laura Silva
    The Sawyer School
    Pawtucket, RI
Pamela Smith
    Private Medical Practice
    Harrisburg, PA

Bruce Sundrud
    Harrisburg Area Community
    College
    Harrisburg, PA
Ann Sugarman
    Berdan Institute
    Totowa, NJ
Dan Tallman
    Northern State University
    Aberdeen, SD
Jackie Trentacosta
    Galen College
    Fresno, CA
Fred Ann Tull
    Southern Technical College
    Little Rick, AR
Deborah Wood
    Concorde Career Institute
    Lauderdale Lakes, FL

And finally, those who gave detailed feedback on our questionnaires helped configure the kit in its present form:

Theresa Bowser
    Southern Ohio College
    Columbus, OH
Elaine Chamberlin
    Pontiac Business Institute
    Oxford, MI
Thelma Clavon
    Rutledge College
    Columbia, SC
Leslie Fiore
    Kentucky College of Business
    Florence, KY
Diane Franks
    National Career College
    Tuscaloosa, AL
Tony Gabriel
    Watterson College
    Pasadena, CA
Karen Greer
    Sawyer College
    Merrillville, IN
Joyce Hill
    Lansdale School of Business
    North Wales, PA

Roxanne Hold
    Excel College of Medical Arts
    and Business
    Madison, TN
Annette Jordan
    Phillips Business College
    Lynchburg, VA
Martha Juenke
    American Medical Training
    Institute
    Miami, FL
Richard Krafcik
    Sawyer College
    Cleveland Heights, OH
Akeeboh Moore
    CareerCom College of
    Business
    Oakland, CA
Basil Punsalan
    Commonwealth College
    Norfolk, VA
Alta Belle Roberts
    Metro Business College
    Rolla, MO

Sharon Adams
    Sasser Sawyer College
    Merrillville, IN

Joyce Shuey
    Academy of Medical Arts and
    Business
    Harrisburg, PA

Mary Ellen Stevenback
    Lansdale School of Business
    Harleysville, PA

Jinny Taylor
    Academy of Medical Arts and
    Business
    Harrisburg, PA

Edith Watts
    Watterson College
    Oxnard, CA

USING THE REVISED MEDICAL ASSISTANT KIT

The 10 anatomy and physiology books form the basis for a one-, two- or three-term introduction to body structure and function and human disease. Each book stands alone and may be used in the most appropriate sequence for your program.

Laboratory Processes for Medical Assisting and *Clinical Processes for Medical Assisting* can supplement the anatomy and physiology books as lab sections or they can be offered as separate courses.

We hope instructors and students alike will find a certain new clarity and precision in this new edition of the REGENTS/PRENTICE HALL MEDICAL ASSISTANT KIT. We look forward to your comments.

Mark Hartman
Editor, Health Professions

The Language of Medicine

As you study this book, you will add new words to your medical terminology vocabulary. Once again, you will find that both Latin and Greek words and word parts are used to name organs, diseases, and medical procedures. You will see that sometimes both Greek and Latin words for the same organ appear in medical terminology; it's helpful to know that differing words or word parts may refer to the same thing.

ren + al (a Latin suffix meaning having to do with)

But your textbook also mentions *nephritis,* from the Greek.

nephr(os) = itis (Greek for inflammation)

And you may encounter the word *nepehrectomy.*

neph(os) + ectomy (Greek for cutting out an organ or gland

Both Latin and Greek have words that mean bladder. The Greek word is *kystis* (Greek *ks* often become *cs* in English) and it appears in many words that have to do with bladder problems and treatment.

cyst + algia (Greek for pain)
cyst + o + scope (Greek, *skopien,* to examine)
cyst + itis

The Latin word for bladder, *vesica,* does not appear in this book, but you may find it elsewhere in medical literature:

vesic(a) + otomy (Greek for cutting into)

meaning an incision into the bladder. Another version of this Latin word does appear in your text, however; it is the name of part of the male reproductive system: the *seminal vesicle.* The suffix *-cle* is a Latin word part meaning little; a *vesicle,* then, is a little bladder (container). The other part of this name comes from the Latin word for seed (and the seminal vesicle contains the sperm, which can be thought of as seeds).

sem(en)in + al vesi(ca) +

Another example of more than one word for the same thing is the Latin word *testis,* the word for the male *gonad,* or sez gland (gonad from the Greek *gone,* meaning seed). The word for testis in Greek is *orchis.* And while your textbook talks about the *testes* (plural of testis), it also talks about such conditions as *orch(is) + itis*

and such surgical procedures as

orchi(s)o = pexy (Greek for a surgical fixation)

and a structural problem called *cryptorchidism*

crypt(o) (Greek for hidden) + *orch(is)* + *ism* (a suffix meaning condition)

You may want to look in the glossary to see if the definition of cryporchidism makes sense when you remember the word parts this word uses. However, *orchis* is not the only Greek word for testis--just as English uses both *testis* and *testicle* for the same thing. Another Greek word for testis is *didymus*, a word that also means *twin*. (Since there are two testes, that meaning makes sense). Forms of *didymus* appear in this textbook in such words as

epi (Greek for *on* or *upon* + *didymis*,

which describes a structure of the reproductive system located on top of the testis. If you pay attention to the words your textbook uses, and make sure that you look up new words in a medical dictionary, your vocabulary of the language of medicine will continue to expand.

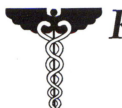 *Knowledge Objectives*

After completing this chapter, you should be able to:

- name the organs that make up the urinary system
- describe the size, shape, position, and function of the kidneys
- name the parts of the nephron
- trace the circulation of blood in the kidneys
- describe the size, shape, position, and function of the ureters, bladder, and urethra
- state the normal amount and content of urine voided daily
- describe the three steps in urine formation
- state the mechanism and substances involved in glomerular filtration
- explain the renal threshold
- describe the mechanisms and substances involved in tubular reabsorption and tubular secretion
- explain how the body maintains fluid, electrolyte, and acid-base balance

Male and Female Urinary Systems

INTRODUCTION

The urinary system has two major functions: the elimination of wastes, and the maintenance of fluid and **electrolyte balance (ee LECK troh lyt)** in the body as a whole. The **kidneys (KID neez)** are the main working organs of the system (see Figure 1). They form the **urine (YOOR in)** by filtering blood. Urine is the solution that remains in the urinary system at the end of this process. The **ureters (yoo REE turz)** convey the urine from the kidneys to the **bladder (BLAD ur)**. The bladder stores the urine until it builds up enough volume to be excreted. The **urethra (yoo REE thruh)** is the passage by which the urine leaves the bladder and exits the body.

The urinary system is one of the few body systems that differ significantly between males and females. The kidneys, ureters, and bladder have essentially the same function in both sexes. The urethra differs between the sexes: In the female, the urethra is relatively short and its only function is to excrete urine. In the male, the urethra is much longer and it has two functions—excretion of urine and ejaculation of semen (a reproductive function).

The first step in understanding how the urinary system works is to look at the system as a whole, and its physical relationship to other body systems. Then we will go into the details of its functions.

URINARY SYSTEM ANATOMY

The two kidneys are found behind the abdominal cavity, outside the **peritoneum (PERR ih toh NEE um;** the membranous sac that lines the abdominal cavity). They lie between the twelfth thoracic vertebra and the third lumbar vertebra, on either side of the spinal column. The ascending section of the colon is in front of the right kidney, and the descending colon is in front of the left one. Part of the liver is above and in front of the right kidney and part of the stomach and spleen is above and in front of the left one (see Figure 1).

The kidneys are shaped like kidney beans. They are oval and rounded, but have a concave area on the edge toward the midline. The center of the concave area is called the **hilus (HY lus)**. Each kidney is 10 to 12 cm long, 5 to 7 cm wide, and 2.5 cm thick.

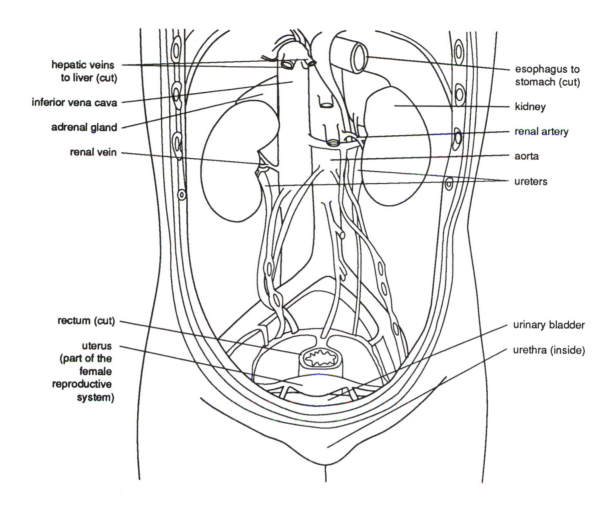

Figure 1: The urinary system. The kidneys lie behind the abdominal cavity outside the peritoneum.

Each kidney weighs approximately 150 gm. The left one is usually slightly larger than the right.

One of the pair of **adrenal (ah DREE nul) glands** sits atop each kidney (see Figure 1). These endocrine glands are discussed in the book on endocrinology in this series. Each kidney and its attached adrenal glands are surrounded and protected by a layer of adipose (fatty) tissue.

At the hilus, the renal artery enters the kidney and the renal vein leaves it (see Figure 1). Also at the hilus, the ureters leave the kidneys. The ureters are narrow tubes leading from the kidneys to the bladder. The bladder is located in front of the rectum and behind the pubic bone.

The urethra is a single tube that leaves the bladder at the lower end. In the female, it leads directly from the bladder to the **urinary meatus (YUR ih ner ee mee AY tus),** an opening just in front of the vaginal opening (see Figure 2). In the male, the urethra passes though the center of the doughnut-shaped prostate gland and then along the entire length of the penis. The urinary meatus in the male is in the center of the tip of the glans penis (see Figure 3).

Kidneys

The outside of each kidney is encased in a tough, fibrous material. If you cut a kidney in half lengthwise, several structures or areas are visible (see Figure 4). The outer portion is the **cortex (KOR tex).** The inner portion is the **medulla (me DUL luh).** With the

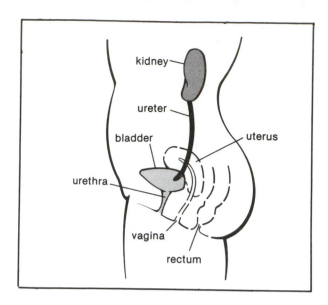

Figure 2: Sagittal view of female urinary system.

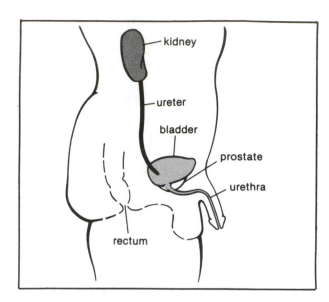

Figure 3: Sagittal view of male urinary system.

medulla are about a dozen triangular structures, the **pyramids (PIRR uh midz)** (see Figures 4 and 5). The tip of each pyramid points inward, toward the hilus. At its tip, the **papilla (pah PIL uh)** (plural; papillae), each pyramid connects with a **calyx (KAY liks)** (plural; calyces), a duct that joins the **renal pelvis (PELL viss).** The renal pelvis serves as a central collection point for urine as it is formed. The ureter for each kidney is attached to the renal pelvis. Between the pyramids in the medulla are sections of tissue called **renal columns**. They are continuous with the cortex, and are made of the same type of tissue as the cortex.

Nephrons. If you take the kidney you have cut in half and look at it under a microscope, you will see its functioning units, the **nephrons (NEFF ronz)** (see Figure 6). There are approximately 1.25 million nephrons in each kidney. Within each nephron are the following structures: A **glomerular (glo MERR yoo lur)** (Bowman's) capsule; a **glomerulus (glo MERR yoo lus),** which is inside the capsule; a **proximal tubule (PROCK sih mul TEW bewl);** a loop of the nephron (Henle), which is a U-shaped continuation of the proximal tubule with a descending limb and an

ascending limb; and a distal tubule. The distal tubule is connected to a collecting tubule, which also is connected to the distal tubules of several other nephrons. The collecting tubules join larger collecting ducts, which carry urine from the nephrons to the calyces and thus to the renal pelvis and the ureters. Each nephron is surrounded by a network of capillaries connected to venules and arterioles, and then to the renal vein and renal artery.

The glomerulus itself is a network of capillaries that feeds into the larger network of blood vessels surrounding the nephron. Together, the glomerulus and the capsule that encloses it are called the renal corpuscle. They are located throughout the renal cortex.

The proximal tubule, loop of the nephron, and distal tubule form a continuous series of tubes in which the urine concentration and chemical content are determined. The loops of the nephron descend into the medulla to the renal pyramids (the descending limb). They return to the level of the renal corpuscle in the cortex (the ascending limb). The cells that make up the walls of each part of this system are slightly different, because each section has its particular role in urine formation.

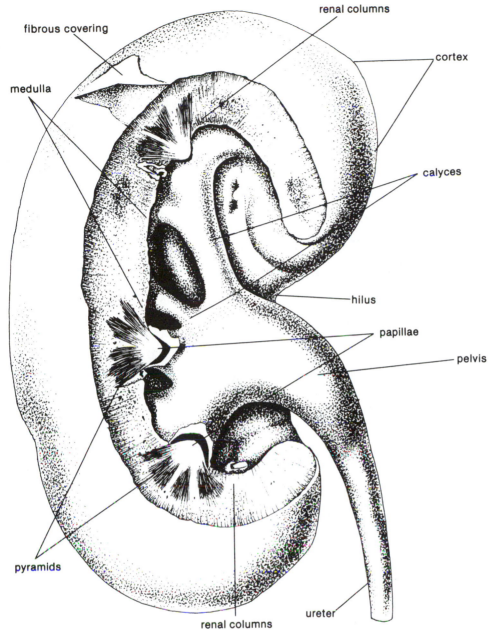

fibrous covering

renal columns

cortex

medulla

calyces

hilus

papillae

pelvis

pyramids

renal columns

ureter

Figure 4: Internal kidney anatomy.

Blood Circulation in the Kidney. Blood enters each kidney though its renal artery. Every minute, the heart pumps about one-fifth of its blood supply to the kidneys through these arteries. Approximately 1,200 ml of blood flows into the kidneys every minute. The renal artery branches into smaller arteries, the **interlobular arteries (in terr LOB yoo lur AHR ter eez).** From each interlobular artery, **afferent (AFF ur ent) arterioles**

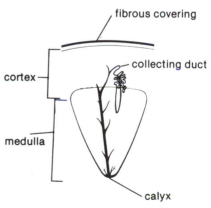

fibrous covering

cortex

collecting duct

medulla

calyx

Figure 5: Pyramids in cortex.

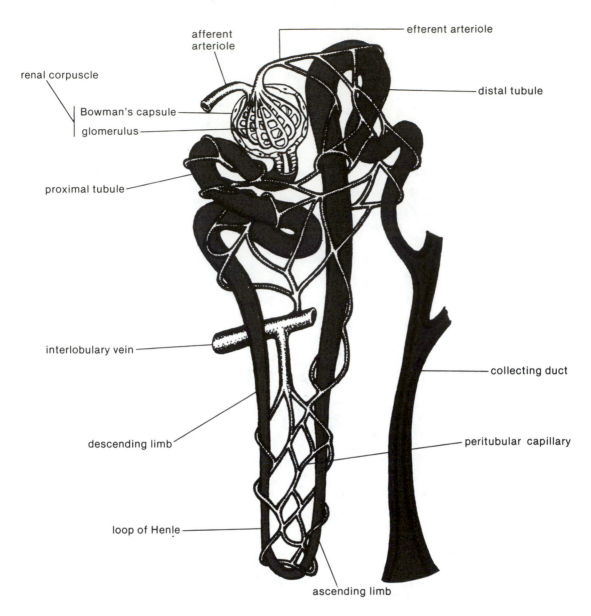

afferent arteriole

efferent arteriole

renal corpuscle

Bowman's capsule

glomerulus

distal tubule

proximal tubule

interlobulary vein

collecting duct

descending limb

peritubular capillary

loop of Henle

ascending limb

Figure 6: The nephron.

(ahr TEER ee olz) carry blood to the renal corpuscles in the nephrons. Inside the glomerular capsule, the arteriole becomes a network of capillaries, which is the glomerulus. At the entrance to the capsule, the **efferent (EFF ur ent) arteriole** drains the glomerulus. This vessel is narrower than the afferent arteriole. This difference in size creates a bottleneck to blood flow in the glomerulus. The bottleneck increases blood pressure in that network, which aids in filtration. The efferent arteriole branches into the network of capillaries that surrounds the entire nephron and reabsorbs fluid and solutes from the tubules. This network, the **peritubular capillaries (per ee TEW bew lur KAP ih lar eez),** leads into a series of larger venules, which join the **interlobular veins**. Those veins lead back to the renal vein, which carries blood out of the kidneys and returns it to the general circulation (see Figure 6).

Before discussing how urine is formed in the nephrons, we will look at the remainder of the urinary tract in more detail, beginning with the ureters.

Ureters, Bladder, and Urethra

Each kidney has a ureter. The ureters are 25 to 30 cm long, and extend from the hilus of the kidney to the bladder along the posterior wall of the abdomen. They have an inner lining of mucous membrane that is continuous from the renal pelvis through the ureters to the bladder wall. The outer wall of the ureters is made up of three layers of smooth muscle. The inner layer is made up of longitudinal muscle. The outer layer consists of circular muscle. The upper third of both ureters has an additional outer layer of longitudinal muscle. Urine is propelled through the ureters by an automatic muscle contraction called **peristalsis (perr ee STALL siss)**. The same type of contraction moves food though the digestive tract.

The ureters enter the lower section of the bladder at an oblique angle. This angle acts as a valve, to prevent urine from flowing back up the ureters to the kidney.

The bladder (see Figure 7) has a mucous membrane lining, which forms into **rugae (ROO gay)** (sing., ruga), or folds, when the bladder is empty. As the bladder fills with urine, the walls stretch and the rugae smooth out to accommodate the fluid. Like the ureters, the bladder is made up of smooth muscle called **detrusor (dee TROO sur)** muscle. The floor of the bladder is triangular and has three openings. The ureters enter at parallel points close to the body of the bladder, and the urethra exits at the bottom of the triangle. At this opening, the smooth muscle changes to form the **internal sphincter (SFINK tur)**. (A sphincter is a circular muscle that surrounds a body opening and causes it to open and close.) Below the internal sphincter is a circle of skeletal muscle, the **external sphincter**. Urination (also called **micturition (mik tyoo RISH un)** or voiding) requires that both sphincters relax. The internal sphincter normally can be con-

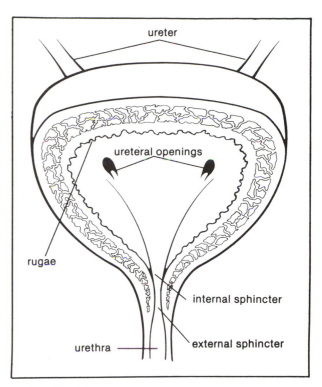

Figure 7: The bladder.

trolled voluntarily, in a child of about age 2; an adult may find it difficult to relax this sphincter when trying to void on demand.

The bladder has a capacity of 350 to 450 ml, depending on the individual (see Figure 8). However, the urge to urinate usually occurs well before it has reached capacity. In most people, 150 to 250 ml of urine in the bladder is enough to stimulate urination.

The urethra is about 4 cm long in the female and about 20 cm long in the male. Like the ureters and the bladder, it is lined with mucous membrane and made up of smooth muscle. The external sphincter is located approximately at the center of the urethra in the female, and just below the prostate gland in the male.

We now return to the kidneys to look at the complex process of urine formation.

URINE PRODUCTION

Under normal circumstances, a person voids about 1.5 L of urine every day. This fluid is

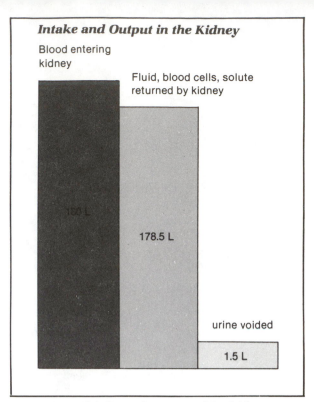

Figure 8: Intake and output of the kidney.

extracted by the kidneys from the approximately 180 L of blood that enter the kidneys daily. Therefore, essentially all of the blood cells and plasma proteins are returned to the bloodstream by the kidneys. Also, about 178.5 L of the original 180 L of fluid and solute are returned to the bloodstream. The content of the urine is regulated by the kidneys, based on a series of chemical and hormonal mechanisms. Normal urine is sterile when it leaves the body, and it contains mainly water, urea, sodium, phosphoric acid, sulfuric acid, and uric acid. Urea is a waste product of protein metabolism, and it is the predominant solute in the urine.

Normal urine contains only a small volume of electrolytes, protein, glucose, and epithelial cells. Blood, hemoglobin, pus, or bacteria exist in the urine only in the presence of urinary system disease or malfunction.

The process of urine formation involves three steps: **glomerular filtration**, **tubular reabsorption** or **resorption**, and **tubular secretion**. During glomerular filtration, a protein- and cell-free filtrate of plasma is filtered from the blood. In tubular resorption, water and solutes are returned to the blood. In tubular secretion, solutes move from the blood directly into the renal tubules.

Glomerular Filtration

Blood from the renal artery flows into the glomerulus and the fluid is filtered out into the glomerular capsule. This fluid is mostly water and also contains solutes—both electrolytes such as sodium chloride and waste products such as urea. The blood cells and plasma proteins remain in the blood vessel, because they are too large to penetrate the membrane.

To understand kidney function, you must first understand some important chemical concepts and terms. Some of these are reviewed in Table 1. If you need further review, reread the appropriate sections in the book on bioorganization in this series.

URINE STUDIES THROUGHOUT HISTORY

Laboratory medicine began with the study of urine. Drawings on cave walls and hieroglyphics in Egyptian pyramids reveal interest in urine as a means of determining the physical state of the body. Some of the first doctors, called "pisse prophets," believed that examining the urine would help treat a patient. Many of the same characteristics were studied then as now: color, odor, volume, and sugar content. Color charts were developed by 1140 A.D., and "taste testing" was common in the late 1600s. By the 1800s, urinalysis was a routine part of a physical examination. Techniques of study and examination have advanced considerably since that time.

Table 1: Review of the Terms and Chemical Processes Involved in Fluid and Electrolyte Balance

1. A **solution** is made up of a fluid called the *solvent*, and other substances that are dissolved in it, called *solutes*. The filtrate in the nephrons is a solution (solvent and solute) called urine.

2. An **electrolyte** is a chemical compound that *ionizes*, or separates into charged particles, in solution. Sodium chloride (NaCl) is an *electrolyte*.

3. **Diffusion**, or spreading, of molecules occurs from a higher concentration to a lower concentration of a substance, or down a **pressure gradient**. Therefore, diffusion of a solute occurs from a more concentrated solution to a less concentrated one. Diffusion of water is also downhill with respect to water concentrations. Water moves *from* a solution with many water molecules and few solute molecules (dilute) *to* a solution with few water molecules and many solutes (concentrated).

4. **Osmosis** is diffusion of water through a selectively permeable membrane in the direction of the greater solutes. The semipermeable membrane selectively allows the passage by diffusion of the solvent (water), but it is impermeable to the solute.

5. **Active transport** across the cell membrane means transport that occurs from the energy released by chemical reactions and is used by living cells. An example is sodium-potassium transport between cells and interstitial fluid, which is assisted by an enzyme. In active transport, the mechanism increases the concentration of the transported substance on the side of the membrane to which it moves. It moves against the concentration gradient (uphill).

6. **Passive transport** includes diffusion and osmosis. It does not require energy from a chemical reaction. Instead, it relies on passive movement of fluids and solutes down their respective gradients through a membrane.

Tubular Reabsorption

From the glomerular capsule, the fluid, or **filtrate**, flows into the proximal tubule, also called the **proximal convoluted tubule** because of its intricate, winding shape. Reabsorption begins in the proximal tubule.

First, sodium moves out of the tubule through the wall of epithelial cells and into the peritubular capillaries. This active transport of sodium creates a difference in concentration between the fluid in the blood vessels and the fluid in the kidney tubule. Approximately 80 percent of the water in the tubule then diffuses by osmosis into the blood to re-establish equilibrium. The tubule wall and blood vessel wall together act as a semipermeable membrane. Some of the solutes, including chloride, bicarbonate, and urea, move into the blood vessels by diffusion.

Glucose and amino acids, which are also in the filtrate in the tubules, move into the blood by active transport, using slightly different mechanisms than sodium. Normally, all these nutrients in the filtrate return to the blood. However, there is a limit to how much can be reabsorbed. This limit is called the **renal threshold**. When this limit is reached, the excessive glucose or other nutrients remain in the tubules and are excreted in the urine.

With this mechanism, medical personnel

can find out, by analyzing the urine, when certain diseases of metabolism are present that cause excess levels of nutrients in the blood. An example is diabetes mellitus, in which the absence of one specific hormone prevents proper utilization of glucose. Excess glucose therefore remains in the bloodstream, and is not available to nourish the cells. The glucose is filtered out in the glomerulus as usual, but abnormal quantities of it are found in the urine—the renal threshold for glucose has been exceeded and not all of it can be reabsorbed.

In the descending limb of the loop of the nephron, sodium continues to be reabsorbed, followed by water, as in the proximal tubule. However, in the ascending limb, the walls of the tubule are different and do not allow water to move through them. Sodium continues to be reabsorbed. Thus, the **osmolality (ahz mo LAL ih tee),** or level of solute concentration, decreases in the ascending tubule and increases in the fluid outside the tubule. The filtrate then continues to flow through the nephron to the distal tubule, and thence into the collecting tubule.

The distal tubule is convoluted, like the proximal tubule. In this part of the nephron, sodium continues to be reabsorbed and water can follow it here; the quantity of reabsorbed water is regulated by **antidiuretic (an teh dye yoo RET ick) hormone** (ADH). ADH is secreted by the pituitary gland and circulates through the bloodstream. (See the book on endocrinology in this series.) How much ADH is released is regulated by the osmotic concentration of the blood.

When ADH is present, the walls of both the distal tubules and the collecting tubules become permeable to water. The extra sodium reabsorbed in the ascending loop of the nephron causes an increase in the number of solute particles in the region of the col-

lecting tubules, thus increasing the reabsorption of water by osmosis from the collecting tubules. This step conserves water. Without ADH, the walls are essentially impermeable to water. To help you remember the effect of ADH, remember that a diuretic drug is one that causes an increase in urination. Therefore, the antidiuretic hormone increases reabsorption of water and causes a decrease in urination.

Water reabsorption is also affected by the hormone **aldosterone (al DOS teh roan)**. If the blood supply to the kidney falls, the kidney releases an enzyme that stimulates the adrenal glands to secrete aldosterone. Aldosterone increases the reabsorption of sodium, which in turn increases the reabsorption of water. This raises the blood volume and subsequently the blood pressure. In this way, the kidney ensures its own continuous blood supply.

Tubular Secretion

The distal tubule is the site of tubular secretion as well as some reabsorption of water and sodium. Secretion is the opposite of reabsorption: substances in the bloodstream move from the peritubular capillaries back into the tubules, to be excreted in the urine. The major substances that enter the urine in this way are potassium and hydrogen, which are secreted by active transport, and ammonium, which is secreted passively by diffusion. Penicillin and other drugs may also be eliminated from the body by being secreted from the blood into the distal tubules.

FLUID AND ELECTROLYTE BALANCE

The amounts of fluid and electrolytes that are reabsorbed in the kidneys vary, depending on need. Regulation of chemical balance

Table 2: Fluid Balance—Intake and Output (*all figures approximate*)

Average daily fluid intake by sources

Drinking liquids:	1000 ml
Eating solid foods:	1200 ml
Metabolism within body:	300 ml
Approximate Total:	2500 ml

Average daily fluid output by mechanism

Urine:	1500 ml
Water vapor from lungs:	350 ml
Fluid in feces:	150 ml
From skin-sweat and diffusion:	500 ml
Approximate Total:	2500 ml

is an essential function—when it fails, the person dies. Intake and use of water and elements such as sodium, potassium, and calcium vary with food intake, exercise, climate, and other factors. To maintain homeostasis **(HOH mee oh STAY siss)**, or steady state, the body needs a regulatory mechanism. The kidneys, working with the endocrine system, supply this mechanism.

Fluid Balance

Let us look first at fluid balance. Water is found in the body in three major areas: the blood; between the cells called **interstitial (in ter STISH uhl) fluid** or **extracellular (ECKS trah CELL yoo lar) fluid;** and inside the cells called **intracellular (IN trah CELL yoo lar) fluid.** It enters the body when liquids are drunk and when solid foods, that contain water, are eaten. For example, an apparently solid food such as a raw cucumber is made up of 90 percent water and 10 percent solids. A small quantity of water is also created within the body by chemical reactions.

Estimates of the quantity of fluid from those sources vary, but normally, fluid intake

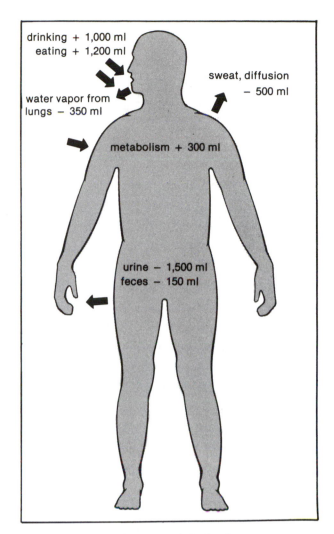

Figure 9: Fluid intake/output of the body.

is balanced by the fluid excretion of four mechanisms, as follows. The most important is urine formation in the kidneys, which accounts for about 60 percent of fluid loss. The other mechanisms are exhalation of water vapor from the lungs, excretion of fluid in feces, and sweating and diffusion of water from the skin surface. Table 2 and Figure 9 show the approximate relationships of fluid intake and output.

Only a single source of fluid intake and a single means of fluid elimination are regulated for purposes of fluid balance. These are drinking of liquids and urination. The **thirst center**, in the hypothalamus **(HY poh THAL oh muhs),** is activated by the volume of blood in circulation and the osmolality of filtrate in the kidneys.

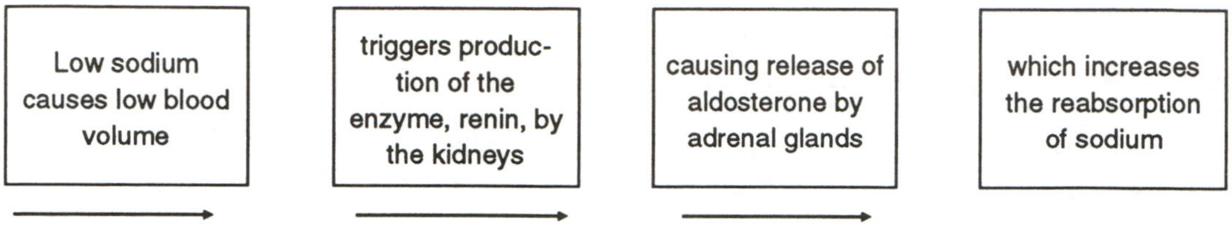

| Low sodium causes low blood volume | triggers production of the enzyme, renin, by the kidneys | causing release of aldosterone by adrenal glands | which increases the reabsorption of sodium |

Figure 10: Sodium balance mechanism.

In the kidneys, as we have seen, fluid excretion is determined by the quantity of fluid reabsorbed in the tubules. The quantity of fluid filtered from the blood remains relatively constant, as does the quantity reabsorbed in the proximal tubules. In the distal tubules, however, reabsorption depends on whether or not the hormones ADH and aldosterone are present. As mentioned earlier, these hormones increase reabsorption and decrease urine output. This mechanism thus retains fluid by returning more water from the kidney tubules to the blood and from there to the cells and the spaces between the cells.

Electrolyte Balance

Electrolyte levels including sodium, potassium, and calcium are regulated by the kidneys.

Sodium and Potassium Balance. We will look first at sodium and potassium, because their levels are influenced by aldosterone secretion. Because the level of sodium directly affects blood volume and pressure, the feedback mechanism for aldosterone which controls sodium reabsorption is based on blood pressure to the kidneys, as previously described (see Figure 10).

The same mechanism, aldosterone release, also influences potassium reabsorption. Ordinarily, almost all of the potassium that is filtered out of the blood in the glomeruli is reabsorbed. However, when aldosterone is present, potassium is exchanged for sodium in the blood, and extra potassium is secreted into the tubule and excreted in the urine.

Most potassium is found within the cells, and the intake of this element usually does not vary. When the kidneys do not excrete sufficient potassium, extra potassium circulates and causes an imbalance. If too much is excreted, a shortage exists. Either condition can cause illness. Causes of and treatment for **hyperkalemia (HY per kah LEE mee uh)** (excess potassium) and **hypokalemia (HY poh kah LEE mee uh)** (not enough potassium) are discussed in the following chapter.

Calcium Balance. Calcium is the major bone-hardening mineral and a vital electrolyte. It is also necessary for muscle function, blood clotting, and transport of materials though cell membranes. A certain level of calcium circulating in the blood is necessary for these functions to continue. The calcium level in urine is regulated by the hormone **parathormone (PAR uh THOR moan),** or **parathyroid hormone (PAR uh THY royd HOR moan),** secreted by the parathyroid gland. The presence of this hormone causes an increase in calcium reabsorption from the tubules to the blood. The calcium is then available for use in bone repair, muscle contraction, and other vital functions. If the proper level of calcium is not returned to the blood, muscle spasms and weakening of bones will follow (see Figure 11).

ACID-BASE (pH) BALANCE

The blood has a normal pH of 7.35 to 7.45.

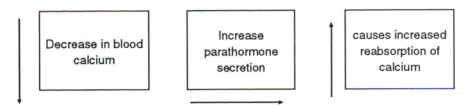

Figure 11: Calcium balance mechanism.

This means that it is slightly alkaline, or base. A base compound is one that releases hydroxyl ions in solution (OH-). An acid is a compound that releases hydrogen ions in solution (H+). It is essential for survival that the proper balance of acid and base be maintained in the blood, within this narrow range. Otherwise, the blood could not transport oxygen and nutrients, carbon dioxide and waste (see Figure 12).

The kidneys help to maintain this balance, again in the distal tubules of the nephrons. Two other mechanisms also participate in maintaining blood pH within the necessary narrow range. They are chemical buffers that counteract acids entering the blood and reduce their impact, and respiratory adjustments that change the amount of carbon dioxide.

The kidney mechanism works as follows: When the blood becomes too acid and the pH level drops, the distal tubules secrete extra hydrogen ions from the blood into the urine. At the same time, more sodium ions are reabsorbed into the blood. The acidity of the urine increases (which decreases the pH reading), and the blood returns to its slightly base norm. This renal mechanism is very sensitive but is less immediate in effect than the other mechanisms.

The pH Scale

The acid-base balance, or pH of a substance is rated on a scale of 1.0 to 14.0; 1.0 is totally acid and 14.0 is totally basic. A pH of 7.0 is neutral—neither acid nor base. The chemical reactions of metabolism and the enzymes that speed them up operate best in specific environments. One factor in these environments is pH. The pH level in various parts of the body differs. For example, the stomach is more acid than the mouth. Each organ has an optimal pH that is necessary for the cells in that part to function and maintain the life of the organism.

Normal blood pH is between 7.35 and 7.45. The pH of urine can vary from about 5.0 to about 8.0 because urine is part of the regulatory mechanism that maintains blood pH in its necessary narrow range.

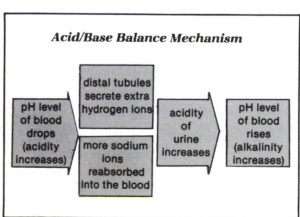

Figure 12: Acid-base balance mechanism.

1. The two major functions of the urinary tract are:

   a. _____

   b. _____

2. The organs involved in #1(a) are: _____

3. The organs involved in #1(b) are: _____

4. Before moving down the ureter, urine is stored temporarily in the _____

5. The automatic, wormlike muscle contraction that propels urine through the ureters is called _____.

6. The bladder is constructed with _____ on its inner mucous membrane that allow it to expand to hold urine.

7. In most people, the amount of urine in the bladder that stimulates micturition is _____.

8. The amount of urine voided daily is normally about _____.

9. The urine voided daily is extracted from the approximately _____ of blood that the kidneys filter daily.

10. Urine formation has three steps:

    a. _____

    b. _____

    c. _____.

11. Fluid filtered from the renal artery into Bowman's capsule contains: _____
    _____

12. _____ move(s) out of the proximal tubule by active transport.

13. _____ move(s) out of the proximal tubule by osmosis.

14. _____ move(s) out of the proximal tubule by diffusion.

15. The amount of water reabsorbed in the distal tubules is regulated by _____ , which is secreted by the pituitary gland.

16. The hormone _____ is secreted by the adrenal glands, in response to the secretion of the enzyme _____ by the kidneys.

17. Substances secreted into the urine by the distal tubules include _____ .

18. Water is found in the body in the:

    a. _____

    b. _____

    c. _____

(continued next page)

19. Average daily fluid intake is _____, and output is _____ .

20. Fluid is supplied to the body by _____ , _____ , _____ , _____ , _____ .

21. Fluid leaves the body in the _____ , _____ , _____ , _____ .

22. Sodium and potassium are involved in the _____ and fluid balance of the body.

23. Sodium and potassium reabsorption are influenced by the presence of the hormone _____ , released from the adrenal cortex.

24. The hormone that controls calcium balance in the blood is called _____ .

25. Acid-base balance in the body is maintained by the:

   a. _____

   b. _____

   c. _____

True or False

26. _____ The fibrous material on the outside of the kidney is the medulla.

27. _____ The opening of the ureters into the bladder is called the internal sphincter.

28. _____ ADH increases urination by decreasing the reabsorption of water.

Circle one

29. Excess potassium in the blood can cause an illness called hyperkalemia/hypokalemia.

30. Blood is normally slightly acid/alkaline.

31. Blood enters the kidney through the renal artery and leaves through the renal vein. Between these two points it passes through the (list the following parts in order):

   _____ interlobular arteries

   _____ afferent arterioles

   _____ peritubular capillaries

   _____ efferent arterioles

   _____ interlobular veins

(continued next page)

32. In the following list, circle the names of the substances contained in normal urine:

water	ammonium	chloride	sulfate
glucose	sulfuric acid	phosphate	blood cells
uric acid	amino acids	ascorbic acid (vitamin C)	sodium
calcium	electrolytes (Cl−, Na+, K+)		creatinine
urea		potassium bicarbonate (HCO3−)	phosphoric acid
protein	hemoglobin		

33. Print the appropriate letters on the following list in position on the accompanying diagram:

   a. Kidneys

   b. Bladder

   c. Ureters

   d. Urethra

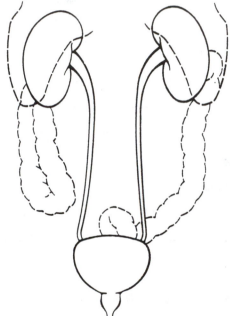

34. Print the appropriate letters on the following list in position on the accompanying diagram:

   a. Cortex

   b. Medulla

   c. Calyx

   d. Hilus

   e. Pelvis

   f. Pyramid

   g. Papilla

   h. Renal column

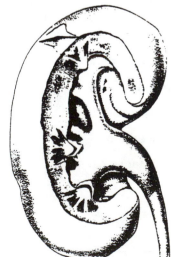

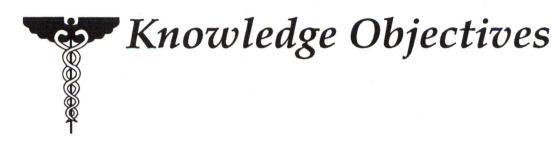

Knowledge Objectives

After completing this chapter, you should be able to:

- describe three special tests and procedures used to diagnose and treat urinary tract diseases
- describe the causes, symptoms, and treatment of some infections of the upper and lower urinary tract
- describe the causes, symptoms, and treatment of some urinary tract obstructions
- describe the causes, symptoms, and treatment of acute and chronic kidney failure

Diseases of the Urinary Tract

This chapter describes some of the best-known and most common urinary tract disorders, along with diagnosis and treatment of those disorders. In women, urinary tract infections generally are not dangerous unless they are neglected or the woman is pregnant. In men, urinary tract infections are uncommon. They are almost always a sign of a more serious problem, such as an obstruction in the system. In children, urinary tract infections are both uncommon and serious. If not treated promptly, they can lead to chronic problems related to infection and kidney damage. One type of infection, sexually transmitted disease (STD), can affect the urinary tract as well as the reproductive system.

Other disorders of the urinary system include stones, cysts, tumors, and various degrees of kidney failure. Injuries to the urinary tract are not common. The kidneys and ureters usually heal quickly, whereas an injury to the bladder may be more serious because of urine leakage into the abdominal cavity and the resulting risk of serious infection.

SPECIAL TESTS

A number of tests and procedures are used to diagnose and treat urinary tract problems. Several of the most common tests are described below.

Urinalysis (yoo rih NAL ih sis) is a basic laboratory examination of the urine. It includes testing for specific gravity (urine concentration), observing the urine to determine color and clarity, basic chemical testing with a dipstick (for glucose, protein, and pH, to name a few), and microscopic examination of urine sediment. These basic tests can be done in the doctor's office and provide essential information about kidney function. Urinalysis findings can be followed up with more detailed chemical tests if necessary. Table 3 summarizes the most common findings. You will learn to perform these tests in the urinalysis section of the laboratory processes book in this series.

Urine culture is done when an infection is suspected and also as a routine precaution in children and pregnant women. A clean-catch–midstream specimen of urine is

Table 3: Urinalysis Findings (continued next page)

| | General Examination | |
Elements	Normal Findings (SI Values)	Abnormal Findings
Color	Pale yellow to deep gold	Color may vary with fluid intake and output or medication; brown or black color indicates serious disease process.
Odor	Aromatic	Fetid odor may indicate infection; fruity odor may be found in diabetes mellitus, dehydration, or starvation; other odors may be due to medication.
Appearance	Clear	Cloudiness may reflect infection.
Specific gravity	1.001–1.030	Concentrated urine has a higher specific gravity. Dilute urine, found in diabetes mellitus, acute tubular necrosis or salt-restricted diets, has a lower specific gravity.
pH	5.0–8.0	pH lower than 7.0 (basic or alkaline) is common in urinary tract infections, metabolic or respiratory acidosis, diet high in fruits and vegetables, or administration of drugs like sodium bicarbonate or potassium citrate. pH higher than 7.0 (acidic) is common in metabolic or respiratory acidosis, fever, phenylketonuria, high protein diets, and ingestion of ascorbic acid.
Protein	Negative to trace	Protein may indicate glomerulonephritis or pre-eclampsia in a pregnant woman.
Glucose	None	Small amounts of glucose may be present as result of eating a high carbohydrate meal, stress, pregnancy, ingestion of some mediations (such as corticosteriods or aspirin). Higher levels may indicate poorly controlled diabetes, central nervous system disorders, Cushing's syndrome, or infection.
Ketones	None	Presence of ketones may indicate poorly controlled diabetes, dehydration, starvation, or ingestion of large amounts of aspirin.
Occult blood	Negative	Occult blood may indicate some anemias, ingestion of anticoagulants (blood thinners), arsenic, poison, or reactions to transfusion, also found in trauma, burns, and convulsions.
	Microsopic Examination	
WBCs	0-5/hpf (high-power field)	Higher levels of WBCs may indicate urinary tract infection.
RBCs	0-5/hpf	Higher levels of RBCs may indicate kidney stones, tumor, or acute glomerulonephritis.

needed; this procedure eliminates bacteria normally found around the urethral opening. A culture plate with an appropriate culture medium is inoculated with the specimen and incubated, usually for 24 hours. Then the bacteria that grow out (if any) are counted and identified. At the same time, an **antimicrobial susceptibility test** may be done. In this test, discs saturated with various antibiotics are placed on the culture

Table 3: Urinalysis Findings (continued)

	Chemistry		
Elements	Reference Range (SI values)	Minimal Quantity Required	Clinical Significance
Creatinine clearance	15–25 mg/kg of body weight/day (0.13–0.22 mmol/kg/day) (Serum creatinine clearance should be determined sometime during the urine collection period)	2,12, or 24 hr	Creatinine may be increased during tetanus or salmonella infection. Decreased with impaired glomerular filtration rate, anemia, leukemia, or muscle atrophy.
Osmolality	50–1400 mOsm/kg (same) 300–900 mmol/kg (same)	Random 24 hr	Osmolality may be decreased with diabetis mellitus; increased with low blood volume.

plate with the specimen to see which ones are effective against the disease-causing organism in the urine. To ensure accurate interpretation, the culture plate must be marked with the name of any antibiotic the patient may be taking.

The **creatinine (kree AT i nin) clearance test** is a more sophisticated laboratory test that is usually done by a commercial laboratory rather than in a doctor's office. A spectrophotometer is used for this test. A 24-hour specimen of urine is mixed thoroughly and a portion of it is tested to learn how much creatinine has been excreted by the kidneys during that time period. This is one way to determine how efficiently the kidneys are functioning. The test is also called a **urine creatinine test**.

For more information on these tests, and details on how they are performed, see the chapter on urinalysis in the book on laboratory processes, in this series.

SPECIAL EQUIPMENT AND PROCEDURES

Catheter

A **catheter (KATH uh ter)** is a tube used in both diagnosis and treatment of urinary tract problems. There are many different types of catheters, made of various materials and in various shapes and sizes. They have three basic uses: to remove urine from the bladder for testing, either to avoid the possibility of a contaminated specimen or to obtain a specimen in a patient who cannot urinate normally; to remove urine from the system in a patient who cannot void for any reason; and to treat **stricture (STRICK cher)** (narrowing) of passageways in the system.

An **indwelling catheter** is one that is implanted in the patient for a time to replace the normal passageway for urine. Any type of catheter, and especially the indwelling type, carries a risk of infection. The catheter should be inserted in as sterile a situation as possible, taking every precaution against contamination.

Cystoscope

A **cystoscope (SISS toh SKOHP)** is a flexible tube having a light source and lens system that is designed for viewing the inside of the urethra and bladder (see Figure 13). The patient is sometimes given a general anesthetic, and the tube is inserted through the urethra into the bladder. With this technique it is possible to observe obstructions, growths, and other abnormalities of the bladder and urethra.

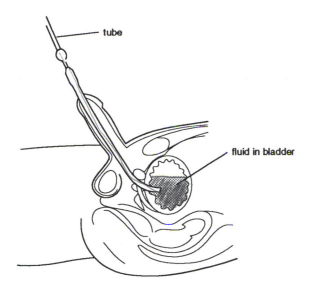

tube

fluid in bladder

Figure 13: Cytoscopic examination.

Cystography

Cystography (siss TOG rah fee) is a procedure in which a radiopaque solution is injected into the bladder and x-ray pictures are taken of it. The solution fills the bladder and may show reflux (the abnormal backing up of urine into the ureters), injuries, or diverticuli.

Sound

A sound is used to treat stricture or obstruction of the urethra. It is a metal rod that is curved at one end and has a handle at the other end. Sounds are available in various sizes (diameters) and are usually about 27 cm (10.5 in) long—more than enough to extend the entire length of the male urethra. The curved tip of the sound is inserted into the urinary meatus and gently passed into the urethra until it reaches the bladder or is stopped by an obstruction or stricture. Insertion must be done with great care to avoid injuring the wall of the urethra. The procedure is usually uncomfortable for the patient, especially when the sound passes through the prostatic portion of the urethra.

Intravenous Pyelogram

An intravenous pyelogram is an x-ray procedure used to visualize kidney function and to detect stones, tumors, obstructions, and strictures. A dye is injected into the patient's veins, and the progress of the dye through the kidneys is photographed in a series of x-ray films. The test requires several hours, but usually is painless.

Kidney Dialysis

Kidney dialysis is kidney function through artificial means. It can be accomplished by one of two methods. The first method uses an artificial kidney outside the patient's body or inside the peritoneal (abdominal) cavity. This method is called hemodialysis **(HEE moh dye AL uh siss)**. Some of the patient's blood is diverted temporarily into a machine that performs the filtering and reabsorption functions of the kidney, then returns the blood to the patient.

The second method is called peritoneal dialysis **(per ih toh NEE uhl)**. In this method, a solution called dialysate **(dye AL ih sayt)** is injected through a catheter into the peritoneal cavity. The peritoneal membrane serves as a kidney membrane, and the exchange of fluid and electrolytes occurs across it. The fluid is removed after about 5 hours and replaced with fresh solution. The solution removed contains the waste materials that would normally be excreted in the urine.

These dialysis techniques are not quite as efficient as normal kidneys, but they can maintain fluid and electrolyte balance for many years in a patient whose kidneys are not functioning. There are side effects and problems associated with both types of dialysis.

Kidney Transplantation

Kidney transplantation can be done in some

cases of kidney failure. The transplanted organ can be taken from an accident victim or a person who has died of a disorder unrelated to the kidneys. The kidney can also be taken from a relative of the affected person because one kidney can perform the work of both if necessary. In either case, the transplanted organ is matched as closely as possible to the tissue type (similarly to the blood type) of the patient. Organs from close relatives are most likely to match well.

The major risks related to transplanted kidneys are rejection of the foreign tissue by the body, and infection. To prevent rejection, drugs that suppress the immune system are given to the patient. This in turn makes the patient susceptible to infection, even from organisms that would not ordinarily cause disease. A delicate balance must be maintained in treatment to avoid both of these dangers.

There are several other terms you should know that relate to urinary tract disorders. **Dysuria (dis YOO ree uh)** means painful urination. **Hematuria (HEE muh TEW ree uh)** means blood in the urine. **Oliguria (OL ig YOO ree ah)** refers to insufficient urine excretion; **anuria (ah NYOO ree ah),** to a complete lack of urine excretion, and **polyuria (POL ee YOO ree ah),** to excess urine excretion. **Pyuria (PY YOO ree ah)** describes the presence of pus in urine. **Nocturia (NOCK TEW ree ah)** describes excessive urination at night. A **cast** is a tiny, cylindrical bit of material formed in the tubules from protein combined with other elements. Most casts indicate the presence of a kidney disease or malfunction if they appear in the urine.

URINARY TRACT INFECTIONS

Urinary tract infections are classified as upper and lower tract infections. Lower tract infections include **urethritis (YOOR eh THRY tiss)** (infection of the urethra) and **cystitis (siss TYE tiss)** (bladder infection). Upper tract infections affect the kidneys. They include glomerulonephritis **(glo mer yoo lo neph RYE tis)** and pyelonephritis **(pye uh lo ne FRY tis)**. It is sometimes difficult for the physician to determine which part of the system is infected, because the symptoms are not completely reliable. Nor are other tests completely reliable. Some physicians follow a policy of treating for a lower urinary tract infection first. If the problem recurs 1 week after treatment is completed, they follow up with longer-term treatment, as for a kidney infection. Kidney infections can lead to kidney damage, and so are much more dangerous than lower urinary tract infections.

Lower Urinary Tract Infections

Urethritis. Infection or inflammation of the urethra can be caused by sexually transmitted infections, such as chlamydial infection (nonspecific urethritis, NSU) or gonorrhea. In a woman, it can be caused by sexual intercourse, especially if she is having her first sexual experience. Sometimes called "honeymoon cystitis" for this reason.

In a man, the symptoms of urethritis are burning pain during urination and a thick, yellowish discharge from the penis. In a woman, the symptoms include frequent urination, pain or burning on urination, and blood or an unpleasant odor in the urine.

The doctor will first determine whether bacteria or other organisms are in the urine, through urinalysis and a urine culture. Depending on these findings, an antibiotic may be prescribed. In men, the cause is usually an infection. In women, no bacteria may be found. In such cases, the doctor may recommend that the patient drink water before having intercourse and urinate immediately afterward. A vaginal lubricant may also be suggested to make intercourse more comfortable.

Cystitis. Cystitis, or bladder infection, is common in women and rare in men, mainly because of anatomical differences in the male and female urethras. Remember that the urinary meatus in the female is in front of the vaginal opening and the urethra is less than 2 inches long. It is relatively easy for infection to travel along the urethra to the bladder, from either the anus or the vagina. The anus is the more common source of infection. A normal bacterial inhabitant of the intestines, **Escherichia coli (esh eh RICK ee uh KO lye),** is the most common cause of lower urinary tract infections. This organism may be transferred to the urethra by wiping from back to front after a bowel movement or during intercourse.

In men, the urethra is about 8 inches long, and the opening is far from the anus, at the tip of the glans penis. Cystitis almost always indicates the presence of another urinary tract problem such as prostatitis, benign prostatic hypertrophy, obstruction of the ureters, kidney stones, or kidney infection.

The symptoms of cystitis usually include frequent but scanty urination, pain or burning with urination, blood in the urine, unpleasant odor and/or cloudy urine, and sometimes **urge incontinence (in KON tih nense),** a strong sudden urge to urinate that does not allow the person enough time to reach the bathroom before micturition occurs. Other symptoms may include fever and lower abdominal pain.

To diagnose cystitis, the doctor will want a clean-catch–midstream urine specimen for urine culture and urinalysis. If bacteria are present in the urine at a high level, an antibiotic probably will be prescribed. The patient may also be advised to drink extra fluids. The female patient will also be advised to wipe from front to back after a bowel movement, so as to avoid contaminating the urinary meatus, and to empty her bladder before and after sexual intercourse. The antibiotic may be given in a single large dose, or in many smaller doses for 1 week to 10 days. A follow-up visit probably will be necessary to check the urinary bacterial content. If the same bacterium has recurred, the patient may now have a kidney infection, that is, the bacteria eliminated from the bladder are now moving down from the kidney. Additional tests and treatment will then be necessary.

In men, pregnant women, and children, cystitis points to the possibility of additional problems. Additional tests and follow-up studies may be necessary. Patients who have diabetes or sickle cell anemia are also at extra risk and may require other treatment.

Upper Urinary Tract Infections

Glomerulonephritis. Glomerulonephritis is an infection of the renal nephrons, in particular the glomeruli. Blood and proteins, which normally remain in the blood vessels in the kidney, leak out into the filtrate. This interferes with normal reabsorption, and can permanently damage the glomeruli. The problem can occur as a complication of streptococcal infection, especially in children. This form of the disease is called **poststreptococcal (post strep toh KOCK ul) glomerulonephritis.**

In its mildest forms, glomerulonephritis may cause no symptoms. It may be discovered only because the patient's urine is tested for some other reason. Casts, especially red cell casts, and high protein levels in the urine are indicators of this disease. More severe forms of the disease cause reduced urine flow, blood in the urine, edema (eh DEE muh) (swelling due to fluid accumulation), fever, headache, nausea, vomiting, shortness of breath, and drowsiness.

Glomerulonephritis is diagnosed by examining urine sediment for casts and blood, and sometimes by a biopsy of the kidney. Treatment depends on the cause and severity of the disease. It may include the use of steroid drugs to reduce inflammation, diuretics to eliminate extra fluid, and vitamin and mineral supplements to restore electrolyte balance. Hospitalization may be necessary, especially if widespread damage to the glomeruli leads to kidney failure.

Acute Pyelonephritis. Pyelonephritis is infection of the tissue that surrounds the nephrons. The acute form of the disease usually is caused by a bladder infection moving up the ureters to the kidney. It can occur with any untreated or persistent case of cystitis, but is more likely if there is an obstruction some- where along the urinary tract, or if the valve-like function of the ureters is not effective for any reason.

It may happen that the ureters are attached to the bladder at an unusual angle because of a congenital abnormality. This, and other conditions including pregnancy, can cause reflux of urine into the ureters from the bladder. Acute pyelonephritis can also arise from an infection in the bloodstream, or for no apparent reason.

Acute pyelonephritis causes sudden, severe pain in the sides above the ilium and below the ribs, which is called flank pain. High fever (as high as 40° C or 104° F), chills, trembling, nausea, and vomiting also occur. Dysuria and a constant need to urinate even when the bladder is empty are also common symptoms. The urine may be cloudy or bloody.

Diagnosis requires urinalysis, urine culture, and possibly blood tests. Kidney infection can be confused with severe cystitis, so follow-up for either diagnosis is necessary. A patient who has had pyelonephritis previously or who may be at risk of more serious illness (such as pregnant women, children, and diabetics), may require additional tests once the initial symptoms have been treated. These include x-ray studies or ultrasound scans of the kidneys, an intravenous pyelogram, and cystoscopy to examine the bladder and ureters for the presence of growths or other abnormal findings.

Treatment consists of antibiotics to combat infection, a bland diet with extra fluids, and bed rest. In severe cases, hospitalization and use of intravenous fluids may be necessary. If an abnormal condition is found, it may be correctable with surgery.

Chronic Pyelonephritis.
The chronic form of pyelonephritis may be caused by repeated, undetected urinary tract infections that periodically affect the kidneys. Reflux from the ureters is a common cause of such repeated, relatively mild infections. The bladder is designed to empty completely with each episode of micturition; however, reflux causes some urine to return to the bladder, and this acts as a reservoir for infection. Kidney or bladder stones can also be a source of infection, as they can block the normal flow of urine through the urinary tract.

Chronic pyelonephritis does not cause specific symptoms at first. Gradually, the kidneys become less efficient and waste products begin to remain in the body instead of being excreted in urine. This leads to fatigue, lethargy, frequent urination, itching skin, and nausea.

Diagnostic tests are the same as for acute pyelonephritis. Any urinary tract infection is treated promptly, and related conditions such as kidney stones are identified and treated. Blood and urine tests are done frequently to detect any new infections. In some cases, the physician may prescribe regular doses of an antibiotic for 1 year or more to prevent an identified infection from aggravating the problem and causing kidney failure.

Sexually Transmitted Infections
Two types of sexually transmitted (venereal) infections often cause urinary tract infection. They are **nonspecific urethritis** (NSU) and **gonorrhea (GON oh REE uh)**. These infections are spread through sexual contact. Their symptoms are similar, and they are also similar to symptoms of other lower uri-

nary tract infections. In both sexes, these conditions cause dysuria—pain or a burning sensation on urination. They also cause frequent urination. In men, there is a cloudy discharge from the penis.

The major difference between these diseases is in the causative organism. Gonorrhea is caused by an organism called *Neisseria gonorrhoeae* **(nys SE re uh gahn er RO ee)**. It is a dangerous infection because it can spread throughout the body, starting with the reproductive system and going on to infect the blood and damage bones, joints, skin, and tendons. NSU may be caused by one of several organisms, most commonly a **chlamydia (klah MID ee ah)**. Chlamydia are microscopic organisms that are similar to bacteria except that they are parasites—that is, they require a host organism for survival.

To determine whether the patient has NSU or gonorrhea, tests are done on urine and/or discharge. There is a specific test for gonorrhea organisms. If neither the gonorrhoeae nor any other bacteria are found, the problem is probably NSU. Treatment for either disease is use of an antibiotic that will eliminate the organism identified in the specimen. Like bacterial infections, chlamydial infections respond to antibiotic treatment. However, an effective drug must be selected. Some strains of *Neisserin gonorrhoeae* as well as other bacteria have become resistant to penicillin and other frequently prescribed antibiotics.

Since sexually transmitted diseases are highly contagious, a patient's sexual partner or partners should be tested and treated if necessary. The infection may also have to be reported to public health authorities. Patients are instructed to avoid sexual contact until treatment is completed, so that the disease will not spread. Sexually transmitted diseases are discussed in greater detail in Chapters 4 and 6.

OBSTRUCTIONS: STRICTURES, STONES, CYSTS, AND TUMORS

Obstruction of the urinary tract can be a serious problem, because the entire purpose of the system is to excrete waste fluid. A blockage can cause secondary infection or damage to delicate mechanisms in the kidney, and it also prevents the system from working effectively. Obstructions can occur in many forms. The most common is the formation of stones in the tract. Other possibilities are tumors, both benign and malignant, and cysts. Some obstructions, like strictures, cause narrowing of the involved structures.

Urethral Strictures

Stricture, or narrowing, of the urethra can result from chronic urethritis or other chronic urinary infections, or from injury to the penis. The problem is rare today. Antibiotic treatment usually clears up infections such as gonorrhea, which were a common cause of urethral stricture in the past.

Chronic infection damages cells and causes scar tissue to form around the urethra. The scar tissue may shrink, thus making the passageway gradually narrower. The symptoms include pain, increasing difficulty with urination, and a tendency to have urinary tract infections.

A stricture is best diagnosed by a ureterogram or voiding cystourethrogram. In these tests, an opaque fluid is injected into the urinary tract and x-ray films are taken as the fluid passes through the tract. In this way, any points of narrowing or blockage can be revealed.

Urethral stricture is treated by inserting a series of sounds into the urethra. Each sound is slightly larger than the previous one, which gradually dilates (enlarges) the urethra. The treatment usually is done under a local anesthetic. The patient may be catheterized to remove excess urine from the bladder, and may be given antibiotic drugs to treat existing infection and to prevent possible infection from the use of instruments in the urinary tract. If the sounds are not effective in opening the stricture, surgery may be necessary to remove the scar tissue.

Kidney Stones

Kidney stones, or **renal calculi (KAL kew lye)**, are more common in men than in women, and tend to occur among families. They also are more common in hot weather, when urine is more concentrated (has less fluid) because of fluid loss from extreme sweating. Occasionally, they are caused by an inherited abnormality of blood. Most kidney stones contain calcium and may be due to excess calcium in the blood. There are other types of stones also.

Stones usually form in the renal calyx and remain in the renal pelvis. They form in the following manner: A small bit of matter does not pass through the ureters but remains in the urinary reservoir in the kidney. Over time, it slowly accumulates layers of solutes from the urine, in most cases mainly calcium. Kidney stones can grow as large as 25 mm in diameter. Stones larger or smaller than 5 mm in diameter may remain in the kidney and may not cause problems. However, pieces of stone may break off and travel through the ureter to the bladder, then eventually out through the urethra.

The symptoms of renal calculi vary with the size of the stone passing through the ureter. Very small stones pass through and cause little or no pain. Stones that are large enough to enter the ureters but not large enough to move through them cause **renal colic (KOL ick)**. This is a severe, stabbing pain that makes the patient literally "double over." Other symptoms are nausea and blood in the urine.

Diagnosis of kidney or ureteral stones is best done by intravenous pyelogram, which allows the stones to be seen on x-ray films in most cases. Stone composition is determined by special analysis after one has been obtained by spontaneous passage or by surgery. Kidney damage or infection can be assessed by appropriate chemical and urine tests.

Treatment for a passing kidney stone involves administration of pain-killing drugs. Sometimes drugs that may dissolve the stone are prescribed as well. In rare cases, the stone causes an obstruction in the system, if the pain is extreme, or if infection occurs and cannot be eliminated, surgery may be necessary. The surgeon removes the piece of stone and possibly also any larger stones in the kidney itself. In most cases, however, the physician may use extracorporeal **(ECKS trah cor POH ree al)** shock wave lithotripsy **(LITH oh TRIP see)** (ESWL), a noninvasive procedure in which shock waves are aimed at the stone, causing it to shatter. The smaller particles then can be eliminated in the urine. As an alternative, the physician may treat a large kidney stone with percutaneous nephroscopy and lithotripsy and may treat a ureteral stone via ureteroscopy.

Kidney stones tend to recur. Changes in diet including reduction of protein intake, increased fluid intake, and medications to discourage stone formation may be helpful. Patients who have had this problem should have frequent check-ups to detect potential problems as early as possible. The pain of renal colic is often severe but the long-range danger associated with kidney stones is chronic infection and kidney damage.

Bladder Stones

This condition is less common than kidney stones. Stones similar in composition to renal calculi form in the bladder and usually remain there. The presence of the stone or stones can cause several problems. First, large stones can block the urethra, preventing normal urination. Second, stones can cause abnormally frequent urination because the bladder feels full even when little urine is present. Third, they can block the ureters or cause reflux of urine toward the kidneys. Finally, all of these conditions encourage bladder infection because urine cannot flow freely through the system and tends to stagnate. This provides a favorable environment for bacterial growth.

Bladder stones cause dysuria, hematuria, and abnormally frequent urination. They can also prevent urination or allow urine to flow only in certain abnormal routes. Diagnosis is made by x-ray studies and cystoscopy; usually both are used.

Treatment for bladder stones usually begins with treatment of infection with antibiotics. Then the stones may have to be removed or broken up. This can sometimes be done with the cystoscope, but it may require more invasive surgery.

Kidney Cysts

A cyst **(sist)** is a fluid-filled sac. Cysts appear on the kidneys in two forms: as a single cyst of unknown origin or as multiple cysts caused by an inherited disorder called polycystic kidney disease. Usually, neither form of cyst is dangerous. A single cyst generally causes no symptoms unless it becomes malignant (cancerous), and this rarely happens. In polycystic kidney disease, the patient may have hematuria and may be especially susceptible to pyelonephritis.

Kidney cysts usually are not discovered unless the patient has some other problem and they are found by accident. If the cysts are discovered, the physician probably will want to examine them to be sure they are not malignant. A sample of fluid is removed from the sac by aspiration (with a needle) and tested.

If the cyst is not malignant and is not causing problems, it will not require treatment. The only treatment for a troublesome cyst is removal of the affected kidney, so it is avoided if possible. Still, a patient can function quite well with only one kidney. Especially in patients with polycystic kidney disease, frequent examinations and urinalyses are recommended to detect an infection that may occur as a complication of the disease.

Tumors of the Kidney

Benign (noncancerous) renal tumors can occur but are rare. Two main types of malignant tumors affect the kidney: **hypernephroma (HY per neh FROHM uh)** in adults, and **Wilms' (vilmz) tumor** in children under 5 years of age. The two types are very different.

Hypernephroma. Hypernephroma usually does not cause symptoms until it is well established. It arises at either end of the kidney and gradually displaces tissue, calyces, and the renal pelvis. Eventually, the renal pelvis becomes distorted and surrounds the tumor. The tumor may secrete renin or other hormones. After invading the kidney, a hypernephroma may spread **(metastasize; meh TAS tuh size)** to the renal vein and surrounding blood vessels and lymph nodes. From there, it may spread to other organs.

The first symptom is usually intermittent but severe hematuria, noticeable kidney swelling, or both. X-ray films, ultrasound, computed tomography (CT) scans, and other tests are used to locate the tumor, and a biopsy is done to determine whether it is malignant.

Hypernephroma is not susceptible to radiation treatment. Chemotherapy for any

secondary tumors and removal of the kidney (nephrectomy, **neh FRECK tuh MEE**) are usually necessary. This type of tumor often is not discovered until it is well established, so cure is not common unless the problem is discovered by accident, during investigation of another disorder.

Wilms' Tumor. Like hypernephroma, Wilms' tumor usually does not cause symptoms immediately. Generally it does not invade the kidney as hypernephroma does. Instead, it forms on the surface of the kidney and metastasizes to the bloodstream, liver, lungs, and sometimes brain.

Wilms' tumor usually is discovered when a young child develops a mass in the kidney area, referred to as the flank. Occasionally, there will be symptoms such as weight loss, anorexia (loss of appetite), and vomiting. Blood in the urine is common with this type of tumor. Diagnosis is made by x-ray studies, ultrasound, CT scans, and biopsy.

The treatment for Wilms' tumor is removal of the affected kidney and other affected structures such as lymph nodes, followed by radiation, chemotherapy, or both. If the cancer has spread, the child has little chance of recovery, but if the tumor is removed before it spreads, the chances of recovery are quite good.

Tumors of the Bladder

Bladder tumors may be benign or malignant. They can be caused by exposure to certain industrial chemicals or other carcinogens (cancer-causing agents). Some researchers believe that tobacco smoke, artificial sweeteners, or abuse of phenacetin (an analgesic, or pain killer) contribute to bladder tumors.

These tumors arise in the bladder wall. They extend into the interior of the bladder as well as into the layer of muscle beneath the mucous membrane of the bladder lining. Malignant tumors may then metastasize to the organs and lymph nodes around the bladder.

Symptoms of bladder tumors depend on their location and size. The most common symptom is severe, intermittent hematuria. If the growth blocks the ureters or urethra, it also causes a decrease in urination, and possibly **hydronephrosis (HY droh neh FRO siss),** or excess fluid in the kidney. This causes flank pain. Any obstruction within the urinary tract may also lead to cystitis or pyelonephritis, with accompanying symptoms of dysuria, frequent urination, cloudy urine, fever, chills, nausea, and flank pain.

Diagnosis of bladder tumors is best made by urinalysis and cystoscopy, but sometimes they can be seen on x-ray films. Biopsy is then done to confirm the diagnosis. Sometimes bladder tumors are secondary, having metastasized from primary tumors in the kidneys or ureters, so it is important to examine the entire system for tumors.

Treatment consists of removing the tumor and, if the growth is malignant, the surrounding structures. Usually, this is done transurethrally and followed up with careful observation via cystography and a new urine test, called Q71A. In rare cases, radiation is used to remove the tumor. In some patients, the entire bladder must be removed. If this is necessary, the patient's ureters are connected to a section of small bowel (ileum), which is then brought out to the abdominal wall and exteriorized, thus draining urine from the kidneys.

Patients who have had a bladder tumor require careful lifetime follow-up, because the tumor is likely to recur. Frequent recurrence may require treatment with drugs that are instilled into the bladder to reduce the tumor or prevent further recurrence.

URINARY INCONTINENCE

Urinary incontinence is the involuntary release of urine. Incontinence may range from continual release to a slight trickle on exertion. It is estimated that over 12 million Americans suffer from some degree of incontinence. It is the second most common reason listed for institutionalization of the elderly. Because of the associated embarrassment, the condition leads to increased social isolation.

There are two main categories of urinary incontinence: acute (transient) incontinence, and persistent (established) incontinence. Acute incontinence is temporary, often associated with an acute illness or infection, medications, or psychological disorders. Once the underlying cause is treated, the incontinence resolves of itself.

Persistent incontinence continues after the illness or infection is resolved or the patient has stopped taking the medication that induced incontinence. Persistent incontinence can be classified as stress incontinence, the involuntary release of urine with coughing, laughing, or lifting; reflex incontinence, the release of urine that is not preceded by any urge to void; total incontinence, a continuous leaking of urine; functional incontinence, loss of urine before the person can reach the toilet; and urge incontinence, the release of a large quantity of urine after only a very brief urge to void and usually has the aspect of functional incontinence as well.

Urodynamic studies can help pinpoint the cause and extent of incontinence. Usually, urinalysis and blood studies are also done to evaluate renal function. Treatment addresses the primary cause of the condition. Some conditions require surgical correction while others may be treated with exercise, weight loss, bladder training, medication, or any combination of these.

When the underlying cause is not correctable, the patient will be taught how to use devices to contain the urine. Support groups are also encouraged to help the individual deal with the shame and loss of self-image associated with urinary incontinence.

KIDNEY FAILURE

When kidney damage from any of the diseases discussed becomes severe, it can lead to kidney failure. The problem can also be caused by circulatory disorders or poisons. Kidney failure can be acute or chronic and can lead to end-stage renal disease, which eventually is fatal.

Acute Kidney Failure

Acute kidney failure can be divided into four categories according to its cause. **Prerenal (pree REE nal) failure** is caused by dehydration (from severe diarrhea or vomiting, for example), by collapse of the blood vessels that supply the kidney, or by reduced heart output. **Vascular (VAS kew lar) renal failure** occurs because blood flow to the kidney is prevented by blockage (embolism), a ruptured blood vessel (aneurysm), or severe hypertension. **Intrarenal (IN trah REE nal) failure** is caused by damage to the kidney itself, from infection (glomerulonephritis) or other causes. **Postrenal failure** occurs because of blockage beyond the nephrons in both ureters or in the kidney pelvis in a patient with only one kidney. It can also be due to a renal injury.

The symptoms of acute kidney failure usually include oliguria, an insufficient production of urine. The exceptions are cases in which the mechanisms for concentrating the urine are faulty; that is, the problem has affected the tubules rather than the glomeruli. Other symptoms may include thirst, diz-

ziness, sudden weight loss, back pain, blood in the urine, and sometimes swelling from fluid accumulation in the body.

It is important to learn the cause of acute renal failure before treating it, because treatments will differ. In dehydration, fluid and electrolyte balance must be restored. If cardiovascular problems are the cause, these problems must be treated to restore kidney function. If the cause is infection, the causative organism must be eliminated. In obstruction, the blockage must be located and removed. Diagnosis is based on urinalysis, urine and blood chemistry tests, measurements of urine volume, and evaluation of associated symptoms. Blood urea nitrogen (BUN), creatinine, and BUN/creatinine ratios are especially significant. X-ray studies and scans may be needed to locate blockages in the urinary tract and/or the blood vessels.

Dialysis is sometimes necessary in acute kidney failure to help eliminate excess fluid, sodium, potassium, and other substances from the blood.

Chronic Kidney Failure

Chronic kidney failure is a gradual loss of renal function over time, rather than a sudden loss of function. It can be caused by progressive kidney damage from repeated infections, such as pyelonephritis or glomerulonephritis, or from other chronic diseases, such as diabetes mellitus.

The symptoms of chronic kidney failure are itching, generalized fatigue, forgetfulness, nausea, loss of interest in sex, and peculiar behavior. High blood pressure and rapid pulse and respiration may also occur. The patient may be anemic. Most patients have a personal or family history of kidney problems.

Diagnosis of chronic kidney failure requires tests of urine volume, urine pH, and urine sodium levels, as well as blood chemistry tests (such as serum creatinine and BUN), and other blood tests, x-ray studies of the kidneys, and sometimes a biopsy.

Treatment usually begins with an attempt to control electrolyte balance by restricting protein and potassium in the diet and carefully monitoring sodium, calcium, and phosphate balances. Occasional dialysis may also help keep fluids and electrolytes balanced. Eventually, end-stage kidney disease will occur.

End-Stage Kidney Disease

This disorder is the final stage of kidney failure. It occurs when chronic kidney failure becomes so severe that the kidneys cannot maintain patient function.

Diagnosis of end-stage renal disease is made by carefully following a patient with chronic renal failure. When dietary treatment and drugs are no longer effective, end-stage disease has occurred. The treatment is usually regular dialysis or kidney transplantation.

In some cases, dialysis can be done at home. In other cases, arrangements can be made for treatment at a dialysis center near the patient's home, or when the patient is on vacation or a business trip. Some patients can continue with their usual activities for many years, and schedule their dialysis at night or on weekends. Others require hospitalization or assistance with dialysis. In the United States, much of the cost of this treatment in older persons is covered by Medicare.

Kidney transplantation is done most often in patients who have end-stage renal disease caused by chronic glomerulonephritis, chronic pyelonephritis, or polycystic kidney disease. Transplantation is not possible when active infection or malignancy is present, or when a patient cannot tolerate immunosuppressant drugs due to allergy, hypersensitivity, or other causes. The decision whether to treat a patient with dialysis or transplantation depends on many factors, including the patient's overall health, age, and preference, and the availability of transplantable organs.

DISORDERS OF ELECTROLYTE BALANCE

Hypokalemia (HY per kay LEE mee uh) and **hyperkalemia (HY poh kay LEE mee uh)** refer to the relative level of potassium (K) in the blood. **Hypernatremia (HY per nay TREE mee uh)** and **hyponatremia (HY poh nay TREE mee uh)** refer to the relative level of sodium (Na) in the blood. Hyper- means excess and hypo- means insufficient.

Hyperkalemia

Excess potassium levels (hyperkalemia) can be caused by kidney failure, in which potassium is not secreted from the blood into the distal tubules effectively. Disorders of the distal tubules and adrenal gland disorders that affect aldosterone secretion also can prevent tubular secretion of potassium. Other causes are tissue damage, in which the potassium content of many dead cells is released into the blood at once, and acidosis, which causes potassium to move out of the cells and into the bloodstream. The symptoms of hyperkalemia are irregular heartbeat and muscle weakness.

In mild cases, hyperkalemia is treated by eliminating the cause. In severe cases, calcium, glucose, insulin, or bicarbonate can be added to the blood intravenously to counteract the effects of the potassium excess or speed the return of potassium to the cells. Enemas can also be given to remove potassium quickly from the body.

Hypokalemia

Hypokalemia results from insufficient potassium in the blood. Muscle weakness is the major symptom and can lead to paralysis in severe cases. Other signs are decreased urine concentration and abnormal electrocardiogram (ECG) readings. Causes of hypokalemia are dietary deficiency of potassium, dehydration due to severe diarrhea or vomiting, alkalosis, and use of certain diuretic drugs. These drugs increase urination, which in turn increases the quantity of potassium secreted into the urine.

Potassium depletion is usually treated with an increase in dietary potassium or with potassium supplements. In extreme cases, potassium can be given intravenously.

Hypernatremia

This electrolyte imbalance generally results from a water deficit in relation to the sodium level. Some specific causes of hypernatremia include fluid loss through the skin or lungs in patients with fever, burns, or increased respirations. Other causes are diabetes insipidus, excessive salt intake, and adrenal gland hyperfunction, as in Cushing's syndrome.

The primary symptoms of hypernatremia are confusion, twitching, seizures, and a decreased level of consciousness that may progress to coma. Other symptoms may include increased heart rate, decreased blood pressure, oliguria, thirst, and dehydration.

The physician may diagnose hypernatremia based on the patient's serum or urine sodium level. Depending on the severity of the imbalance, treatment may require administration of salt-free fluids, use of a salt-restricted diet, and limitation of drugs that promote sodium retention.

Hyponatremia

Generally speaking, hyponatremia is caused by a relative excess of body water. It is associated with vomiting, diarrhea, edema, renal failure, certain drugs, syndrome of inappropriate secretion of antidiuretic hormone (SIADH), and other conditions.

This electrolyte imbalance may cause anxiety, headaches, weakness, convulsions, decreased blood pressure, increased heart rate, nausea, vomiting, oliguria, and cold clammy skin.

Low serum and urine sodium levels help identify hyponatremia. Treatment requires correction of the underlying cause of the imbalance; for example, correction of volume deficits, restriction of water intake, or limitation of certain drugs.

Fill in the blanks.

1. A urine test that uses a spectrophotometer and a 24-hour urine specimen is called a

    _____ .

2. A tube for removing and introducing fluids, used for diagnosis and treatment of urinary problems, is a _____ .

3. A tube with a light source and lens used to see the inside of the urethra and bladder is a _____ .

4. The major dangers of kidney transplantation are:

    a. _____

    b. _____

5. Lower urinary tract infections affect the_____ and _____ .
    Upper urinary tract infections affect the _____ .

6. Two causes of urethritis are:

    a. _____

    b. _____

7. _____ and _____ in the urine are symptoms of glomerulonephritis.

8. Give two possible causes of reflux:

    a. _____

    b. _____

9. Give two possible causes of pyelonephritis:

    a. _____

    b. _____

10. Pyelonephritis is diagnosed by means of:

    a. _____

    b. _____

11. Two sexually transmitted infections that can cause urinary tract infection are:

    a. _____

    b. _____

12. Which of the sexually transmitted infections in Question 11 may be caused by parasites? _____

13. Kidney stones are more common in _____ weather because urine is
    _____ when there is more water loss (sweating).

(continued next page)

14. Symptoms of renal calculi that block a ureter are:

   a. _____

   b. _____

   c. _____

15. A kidney malignancy that displaces normal kidney tissue is called a _____ .

16. Symptoms of a bladder tumor can include:

   a. _____

   b. _____

   c. _____

17. The four categories of acute kidney failure are:

   a. _____

   b. _____

   c. _____

   d. _____

   Which of these can involve problems with blood supply to the kidney? _____

18. Gradual loss of renal function caused by repeated infections or by other diseases is also called _____ .

19. Name two treatments for end-stage kidney disease.

   a. _____

   b. _____

True or False.

20. _____ Flank pain is acute, sudden pain in the side below the ribs and above the ilium.

Circle one.

21. Urinary tract infections are most common in men/women/children.

22. Bladder stones are more/less common than kidney stones.

Short Answer.

23. Define the following terms:

   a. Urinalysis _____

   _____

   b. Urine culture _____

   _____

(continued next page)

24. Describe the differences between hemodialysis and peritoneal dialysis. _____
_____

25. Describe the similarities between cystography and an intravenous pyelogram. _____
_____

26. Define these terms:

   a. Cast _____
_____

   b. Dysuria _____

   c. Hematuria_____

27. Cystitis is more common in women than in men because _____
_____

28. Define urge incontinence, and tell what disease(s) may produce it.
_____
_____

29. What structures does glomerulonephritis affect, and how does it affect them?
_____
_____
_____

30. Why is obstruction of the urinary tract a serious problem?
_____
_____
_____

31. Describe the treatment necessary for kidney cysts._____
_____

32. Define oliguria, which is usually a symptom of acute kidney failure. _____
_____

33. How does the physician determine that a patient has end-stage kidney disease?
_____
_____
_____

34. Why is the correct potassium level in the body important?
_____
_____
_____

35. Why can kidney failure cause hyperkalemia?
_____
_____
_____

36. How is excess potassium removed from the body or blood?

_____

_____

_____

_____

37. List three types of incontinence and their symptoms.

a. _____

b. _____

c. _____

Mix and Match.

Place the letter of the special equipment or procedure next to the appropriate definition.

    a. Sound

    b. Catheter

    c. Cystography

    d. Cystoscope

    e. Dialysis

    f. Intravenous pyelogram

38. _____ Metal rod used to treat stricture.

39. _____ Tube with light source and lens system used for examination.

40. _____ Tube for draining urine from the bladder.

41. _____ Removal from the body of soluble substances by diffusion.

42. _____ An x-ray procedure in which opaque solutions are injected in the bladder.

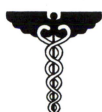 *Knowledge Objectives*

After completing this chapter, you should be able to:

- describe the location, anatomy, and function of the testes, epididymis, vas deferens, seminal vesicles, bulbourethral glands, and penis
- name the male reproductive hormones
- describe the process of spermatogenesis

CHAPTER 3

The Male Reproductive System

INTRODUCTION

The purpose of the reproductive system is continuity of life; it is the sole mechanism by which human life is sustained. The male and female reproductive systems work together to bring this about, but they are quite different. The male produces **sperm (spurm)** and transfers them to the female. The female produces eggs which, if fertilized by the sperm, begin the process of reproduction. (For more information about the female reproductive system, see Chapters 5 and 6.) Sex hormones secreted by the reproductive organs and the pituitary gland are responsible for the maturation and maintenance of the organs as well as secondary sex characteristics and the sexual drive.

Male Reproductive Structures and Organs

In the male, the organs and structures of the reproductive system are located close to the lower urinary tract, and diseases of either system often affect the other. In fact, the two systems share a common passageway to the outside, the urethra, which is inside the penis (see Figure 13, page 23).

The male reproductive system consists of a series of tiny tubes between the testes, where the sperm are made, and the urethra, through which they exit from the body. Along the way are several glands that add fluids to the sperm to aid them in their ultimate goal, the fertilization of an ovum in the female. Though the sperm are formed in the testes, they must mature before they can fertilize an ovum. Therefore, sperm are stored in the system where they mature between the time when they are manufactured and the moment of ejaculation. We will look first at the location and function of the testes, and then, to review the entire system, follow the path the sperm follow.

Testes

There are two **testes (TES teez)** (also called **testicles** [TES tih kulz]), one on each side of the penis and slightly behind it (see Figure 14). The testes are suspended below the body in a sac of loose skin called the **scrotum (SCROH tum).** In the male embryo, the testes are formed in the abdominal cavity, close to the kidneys. They normally move down into the scrotum before birth. Sometimes one or both testes are undescended at birth, a condition called **cryptorchidism (krip TOR**

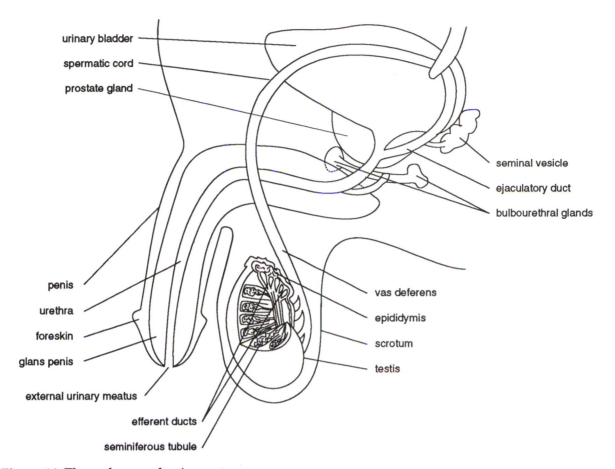

Figure 14: The male reproductive system.

kihd izm). The testes are located below the body for a simple reason. Sperm production, **(spermatogenesis [SPER mah tow GEN ih siss]),** requires a certain temperature range that is slightly cooler than internal body temperature, so the testes are suspended below the body. If the testes become too cool, the scrotum tightens up, thus moving the glands closer to the body's warmth.

The testes are divided into many small areas or lobes. Each lobe contains one or more convoluted tubules, called **seminiferous tubules (SEH mih NIF er uss),** where sperm are made

INTERCOURSE FREQUENCY AND MALE FERTILITY

In men with low fertility, frequent intercourse can increase the chances for fertilizing the female egg. However, too-frequent intercourse may reduce the number of sperm. Most men replenish their normal daily sperm count of 100 to 125 million within 24 hours. In men with low fertility, 3 or 4 days may be required to do this. For every 14 million sperm emptied into the vagina, between 1 and 10 reach the end of the uterine tube. It is untrue that men can abstain from sex for a long time to increase the sperm count. Sperm motility (the ability of the sperm to move) suffers if more than 8 to 10 days elapse between ejaculations. Also sperm production begins to level off after about 5 or 6 days of abstinence.

by a type of cell division called **meiosis (my O siss)**.

The testes also contain specialized cells called interstitial endocrinocytes **(en doh KRIN oh syts)**, which produce the hormone **testosterone (tess TOSS tur ohn)**. This is the major male sex hormone. It stimulates production of sperm and promotes the development and maintenance of male sex characteristics, such as facial and body hair, deepening of the voice, strengthening of the bones, and increased muscle mass. Testosterone is produced throughout life, but production increases just before puberty. It stimulates the maturation of the male sex organs and brings about other body changes related to sexual maturity. This hormone also regulates male sexual behavior, and plays a part in metabolism and urinary tract functions. (Small amounts of testosterone are also produced in women to aid in their metabolism.)

Epididymis

A structure called the **epididymis (EP ih DID ih miss)** is attached to the side of each testis (see Figures 13 and 14). Inside the epididymis is a coiled tubule that, when uncoiled, measures about 6 m (20 feet) in length. The epididymis itself is only about 5 cm (2 in) long. At one end, it is connected to the testis by a network of ducts through which sperm enter. At the opposite end, it leads into the vas deferens. The epididymis serves as a collection and storage center for the sperm.

Vas Deferens and Seminal Vesicles

The **vas deferens (VAHS DEF ur enz)** (plural; vasa) is a tube that leads from the epididymis to the **seminal vesicles** (see Figure 14). Each vas deferens is protected by a spermatic cord, a sheath of connective tissue that also contains blood vessels. These tubes transport the sperm up into the body. They end just below the bladder on either side, very close to where the ureters enter the bladder. They pass through the **inguinal (ING gwi nal)** canals on the way.

The seminal vesicles are located on the underside of the bladder, in front of the rectum. They are pouch-like structures that secrete a thick, yellowish fluid rich in fructose, a simple sugar. This fluid is added to the sperm as they pass through the vas deferens. It forms about 30 percent of the **semen (SEE men)**, the fluid in which sperm are carried.

The seminal vesicles and the vas deferens join below the bladder and within the circle of the prostate gland. From this junction to the top of the urethra are two short ducts called the **ejaculatory (ee JACK yoo loh toh ree) ducts** (see Figure 14).

Prostate Gland

The **prostate (PROS tayt)** is a doughnut-shaped gland located below the bladder and seminal vesicles (see Figures 13 and 14). Inside the "doughnut hole" are the ejaculatory ducts and the beginning of the urethra. The prostate gland secretes a thin, alkaline fluid that is added to the semen. This secretion makes up about 60 percent of the semen. Its purpose is to protect the sperm from acids in the male urethra, through which they must pass as they exit the body, and from acids in the female vagina. Sperm must be motile **(MOH tyl)**, or able to move, in order to reach and fertilize an ovum. They are most motile in a neutral to slightly alkaline environment. So the main purpose of the prostate gland is to ensure a suitable environment for the sperm to do their job.

Bulbourethral (Cowper's) Glands

Just below the prostate gland and about 1 inch from the urethra on each side is a pair

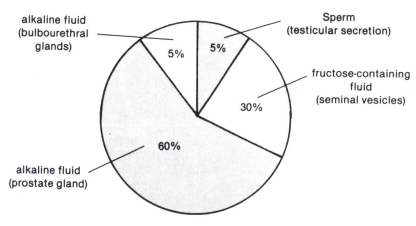

Fluid Composition of Semen

alkaline fluid (bulbourethral glands) — 5%

Sperm (testicular secretion) — 5%

fructose-containing fluid (seminal vesicles) — 30%

alkaline fluid (prostate gland) — 60%

Figure 15: Fluid composition of semen.

Table 4: Summary of Contents of Semen

A milliliter of semen is made up of the following:

- Approximately 70 million sperm (less than 20 million sperm in the semen is considered an indication of male sterility)
- Secretions from the testes, which make up 5% of fluid content
- Secretions from the seminal vesicles, which contain fructose to nourish the sperm cells, and constitute 30% of fluid contents
- Alkaline fluid from the prostate gland, which protects sperm from acids found in male and female reproductive tracts, and constitutes 60% of fluid contents
- Alkaline fluid from Cowper's glands, which forms about 5% of fluid contents

of glands called the **bulbourethral (BUL oh yoo REE thral) glands,** or **Cowper's glands** (see Figure 14). They are very small, each about the size of a pea, and are connected to the urethra by tiny ducts. These glands secrete a fluid similar to prostate fluid, which is alkaline and makes up about 5 percent of the semen. Table 4 and Figure 15 summarize the content of the semen.

Male Urethra and Penis

The male urethra is a tube about 20 cm long that extends from the ejaculatory tubes to the tip of the penis (see Figure 16). It has three named sections: the **prostatic (pross TAT ick)** portion, which is closest to the prostate gland; the **membranous (MEM brayn uhs)** portion, in the middle; and the **cavernous**

(KAH ver nuhs) portion, which passes through penile tissue called **erectile (ee RECK tyl)** or **cavernous tissue** (see Figure 16). The urethra is used for ejaculation of semen and for urination. The muscular action involved in each function "closes off" the other system, so that the two systems operate separately. However, it is quite common to find a few sperm in male urine if it is examined under a microscope.

The **penis** is made up of three separate, parallel cylinders of erectile tissue. This tissue is full of arteries and veins (see Figure 17). When a man is sexually stimulated, the arteries dilate and fill with blood, and the veins constrict. The penis becomes engorged with blood, causing an **erection (ee RECK shun).** The penis becomes larger, longer, and

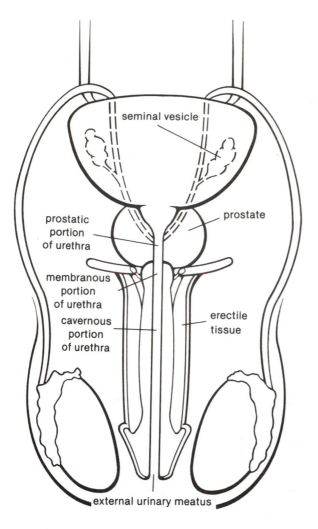

seminal vesicle

prostatic portion of urethra

prostate

membranous portion of urethra

cavernous portion of urethra

erectile tissue

external urinary meatus

Figure 16: Male reproductive organs, anterior view.

rigid. After this, if stimulation continues, the sperm and its accompanying fluids move through the reproductive system into the urethra. This reflex movement is called **emission (ee MISH un)**. After that, automatic muscle contractions along the length of the urethra push the semen though the duct and out of the penis. This is ejaculation. When combined with other signs of sexual response such as accelerated heartbeat, an increase in blood pressure, increased breathing, and dilated blood vessels, ejaculation becomes **orgasm (OR gazm)**, or sexual climax.

The tip of the penis is called the **glans penis** (see Figure 14). It is slightly wider than the rest of the penis, forming a slight bulge at the end. The urethral opening, or **external urinary meatus**, is located there. Over the glans is a loose fold of skin called the **prepuce (PREE pewse)**, or foreskin. This is sometimes removed a few days after birth, in a procedure called **circumcision (sir cum SIZH un)**. Circumcision used to be routine in the United States, but not in some European countries. Today, it usually is not considered necessary and the parents decide whether or not to have their male children circumcised.

THE MALE HORMONAL SYSTEM

As we have seen, testosterone is the main male sex hormone. The male does not have a hormonally controlled reproductive cycle like the female, but does have a system of hormones that regulates testosterone production and thus sperm production.

Testosterone production is controlled by hormones produced in the pituitary gland. The two important ones are **follicle (FOL lih kul) -stimulating hormone (FSH)** and **interstitial cell-stimulating hormone (ICSH)**. These hormones are called **gonadotropins (GON ah doh TROH pins)**. They are also found in women; ICSH is the same as **luteinizing (LOO tee ih NY zing) hormone (LH)**, which plays a role in the menstrual cycle along with FSH. This is discussed more fully in Chapter 5, The Female Reproductive System.

In the male, FSH stimulates sperm production, while ICSH stimulates testosterone production. When the testosterone in the blood rises to a certain level, production of FSH and ICSH is reduced, followed by reduced sperm and testosterone production.

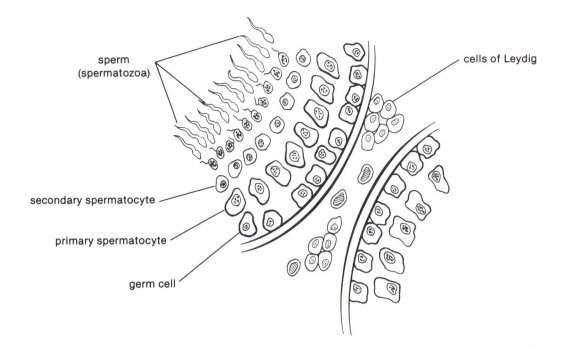

sperm (spermatozoa)

cells of Leydig

secondary spermatocyte

primary spermatocyte

germ cell

Figure 17: A section of the testis showing the development of sperm from the male germ cell to sperm ready for storage in epididymis.

As the testosterone level drops again, gonadotropins are secreted in greater volume, and the cycle resumes. This mechanism is known as **negative feedback**. (It is discussed more fully in the book on endocrinology in this series.)

SPERMATOZOA

Sperm are more formally called **spermatozoa (SPER mah toh ZOH uh)** (singular, spermatozoon). They are formed in the testes by the millions, from meiotic division of male germ cells (see Figure 17). Each spermatozoon has 23 chromosomes—22 autosomal chromosomes and one sex chromosome, either an X or a Y chromosome. When a spermatozoon unites with an

THE EFFECTS OF ANABOLIC STEROIDS ON THE MALE REPRODUCTIVE SYSTEM

The use of muscle-building anabolic steroids by athletes has received much attention. These steroids are derivatives of testosterone and are used to increase muscle mass, endurance, and a "competitive spirit." The justification for their use has been the unfounded belief that because these compounds are manufactured by the body they are safe and "good for you." This is not true. Steroids can be addictive and can cause liver dysfunction, severe infertility, prostate enlargement, and testicle damage. Since the normal production of testosterone occurs by negative feedback, steroid ingestion can affect testosterone production by permanently depressing the manufacture of gonadotropin-releasing factors in the hypothalamus. In female "body builders," the use of steroids not only adds muscle but also alters muscle proportions, as well as secondary sex characteristics, causing such changes as shrinkage of the breasts and uterus and enlargement of the clitoris. In women, the use of anabolic steroids can also lead to irregular menses. Taking these drugs for nonmedical reasons is a violation of the rules of most athletic organizations.

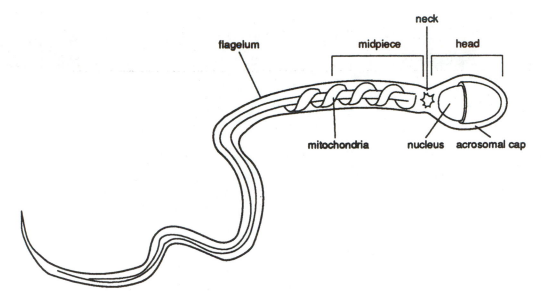

Figure 18: Structure of a sperm.

ovum, they make a single cell having 46 chromosomes. That cell then divides and differentiates to form an embryo. If the sperm has an X chromosome, the resulting newborn will be female. If it has a Y chromosome, the infant will be a male.

The spermatozoa have a unique structure (see Figure 18). At one end is the **head**, which contains the genetic material and mitochondria **(MY toh KON dree uh)**, the cell structures that produce energy. The **acrosome (ACK roh sohm)**, a cap at the tip of the head, produces an enzyme that enables the sperm to penetrate an ovum. The cell nucleus is located directly behind the head in a section called the midpiece of the cell. It also contains mitochondria. The rest of the cell is a long, thin **tail**, which is also called a **flagellum (flah JEL um)**. It lashes back and forth to move sperm through the female reproductive tract and reach the ovum. Of some 14 million sperm cells in a single ejaculation, 10, at most, will penetrate deeply enough into the uterine tubes to fertilize an ovum. However, an ovum may or may not be present in the female reproductive system when intercourse takes place.

STOP AND REVIEW

Fill in the blanks.

1. Testosterone is produced by the _____ . Testosterone stimulates production of _____ .

2. The epididymis is connected to the _____ at one end and to the _____ at the other.

3. _____ move through the vas deferens on the way to the _____ , where a fluid containing _____ is added.

4. The prostate gland secretion added to the semen is _____ , in order to protect the sperm from _____ in the male urethra and _____ .

5. The three named sections of the male urethra are:

   a. _____

   b. _____

   c. _____

6. Movement of semen into the urethra is called _____
   Movement of semen out of the penis is called _____ .

7. Production of testosterone is controlled by _____ ,
   which is produced in the _____ .

8. _____ stimulates sperm production; _____ stimulates testosterone production.

9. The head of the sperm contains _____ and _____ .

True or False.

10. _____ Sperm is stored in the seminiferous tubules.

Circle one.

11. The cell division process that produces sperm is called meiosis/mitosis.

Short answer.

12. The male reproductive system and urinary system are closely connected because _____
    _____
    _____

13. The physical cause of an erection is _____
    _____
    _____

14. What is the negative feedback mechanism? _____
    _____
    _____

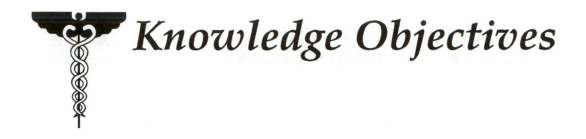

Knowledge Objectives

After completing this chapter, you should be able to:

- list three examinations that are performed to evaluate the male reproductive system
- describe the causes, symptoms, and treatments of three infections of the male reproductive system
- name three sexually transmitted diseases (STDs), and describe their symptoms in men and their treatments
- discuss five ways to reduce the risk of STD transmission
- describe the cause, symptoms, and treatment of three abnormal growths of the male reproductive system
- describe the symptoms and treatment of three cancers of the male reproductive system
- describe the causes, symptoms, and treatments of three structural and three functional problems of the male reproductive system

Disorders of the Male Reproductive System

INTRODUCTION

This chapter covers disorders that are unique to the male reproductive system, and the special instruments, procedures, and tests that are used to diagnose and treat them. As you study this material, remember the close relationship between the male reproductive system and the urinary tract. This is especially important in relation to the prostate gland, which forms a ring around the top of the urethra and often involves the urinary tract when it becomes diseased.

The male reproductive system is subject to the same types of diseases and disorders as any other part of the body: infections, abnormal growths (cancerous and benign), and disorders that affect the structure or function of various parts of the system. Many of the diagnostic and treatment techniques used on the urinary tract are also used to evaluate disorders of the male reproductive system, such as catheters, cystoscopy, and intravenous pyelograms. The resectoscope **(ree SECK toh skohp)** is used specifically to treat problems of males.

A resectoscope is similar to a cystoscope. It is a narrow tube having a light and lens system and an instrument that is used to cut away tissue. The resectoscope is designed specifically to be inserted into the male urethra for the purpose of examining the organs and, when necessary, removing bladder tumors or part of the prostate gland. This procedure, **transurethral resection (trans yoo REE thrul re SECT shun)** is done with the resectoscope.

Prostatic fluid can be examined on a slide using the low-power lens of a microscope. If the gland is infected, pus cells probably will be visible in the specimen. It is also possible to culture the fluid. If a culture is needed, extra care must be taken not to contaminate the specimen. The urinary meatus is thoroughly cleaned with soap and water, and the patient is asked to empty his bladder to eliminate any bacteria that may be in the urethra.

Next we will look at specific diseases of the male reproductive tract.

INFECTIONS

Many different organisms can cause infections in the male reproductive tract. Some of them travel from the urethra to orher parts of the system. Others enter the system through the bloodstream. Also, several genital infections are passed from person to person through sexual contact. Gonorrhea and NSU have been discussed; some STDs that are especially troublesome for the male are discussed next.

Prostatitis

Infection of the prostate gland, or **prostatitis (PROS tah TYE tiss)**, can begin from organisms traveling up the urethra or through the bloodstream. It is not an uncommon disorder, but it is more common in older men who have enlarged prostate glands.

Prostatitis can be acute or chronic. In the acute form, it causes burning on urination, frequent urination, **nocturia (nock TEW ree uh)** (waking at night to urinate), fever, low back pain, painful bowel movements, cloudy urine, and sometimes hematuria or urethral discharge. If the infection develops into an abscess, the abscess may burst and cause a discharge containing blood or pus to flow from the urethra or rectum. The gland also may swell and constrict the urethra, which passes through the center of the gland. This will cause pain and tenderness at the base of the penis, and reduced urine flow.

Prostatitis can lead to bladder or kidney infection since infection tends to travel up the urinary tract. This is especially likely if the prostate gland swells and prevents normal urination. The urine then stagnates in the bladder and harbors bacteria.

The chronic form of prostatitis often does not cause symptoms other than mild discomfort and occasional mild fever. It may lead to **epididymitis (EP ih DID ih MY tiss)** (inflammation of the epididymis) or cystitis.

Diagnosis of prostatitis is made by testing urine and prostate secretions and by rectal examination of the gland. Acute prostatitis will cause bacteria and pus to appear in the urine and prostatic fluid, whereas in chronic prostatitis only pus cells may appear in these fluids. The chronic form of the disease may be caused by chlamydia rather than bacteria, so tests for bacteria will give negative results.

It is important for the physician to avoid use of instruments if possible when the gland is severely inflamed, because the infection may spread or the gland may be damaged. It may be necessary to use a catheter, however, to remove excess urine from the bladder in cases of blockage.

Acute infection is treated with antibiotics, usually penicillin. Chronic infection may occur if treatment does not completely eradicate the causative organism. The chronic form of the infection is more difficult to treat. Carefully chosen drugs that have direct effects on the gland may be helpful. Other measures include regular sexual intercourse for the same reason and hot baths to relieve inflammation. If these treatments are not effective, transurethral resection may be necessary to remove the infected tissue from the gland.

Epididymitis

Epididymitis is closely associated with prostatitis. It sometimes occurs following removal of the prostate gland or prostatectomy **(pros tah TECK toh mee)**, but most often it is a complication of prostate infection. The patient develops a sudden pain in the scrotum. The epididymis swells to twice its normal size within a few hours. Usually the testis also becomes inflamed, but not infected. The patient may have a fever as high as 40° C (104° F).

Epididymitis is diagnosed by the symptoms, palpation of the testes and prostate, urinalysis, and analysis of any discharge from the penis. In a young man, epididymitis can be mistaken for **torsion (TOR shun)** (twisting) of the testis. Epididymitis can also be caused by chlamydia, gonococci, mumps, or bacterial infections from the urine. After appropriate urine tests and cultures, antibiotics and anti-inflammatory drugs are usually prescribed and are often effective when combined with rest and avoidance of irritants, such as alcohol and spicy food. The condition can progress to abscess, and may require surgical treatment.

Sometimes lifting a heavy object or receiving a blow to the testis can cause epididymitis. Bilateral epididymitis can lead to infertility due to scarring of the ducts.

Orchitis

Orchitis (or KYE tiss) is an inflammation of the testes. It usually occurs as a complication of an infection such as mumps in the young adult, after puberty. The symptoms are pain, redness, and swelling of the scrotum around the affected testis, fever as high as 40° C, and prostration. The infection may damage sperm-forming cells and can cause sterility if both testes are affected.

Mumps is a viral disease, so antibiotic drugs are not effective against it. (Most of the other causes of orchitis are also viral.) Therefore, the disease itself cannot be cured, and treatment is aimed at relieving the symptoms. Pain relief, sometimes by injection of a local anesthetic, and bed rest are usually prescribed. Heat or cold applied directly to the swollen testis may provide some relief, and supporting the testes with a padded athletic supporter may also help. The swelling usually lasts 1 week. A few months later, the testes may be noticeably atrophied, or shrunken.

Balanitis

In most cases, **balanitis (BAL ah NYE tiss)** is basically an irritation or infection of the fore-skin or outer surface of the glans penis. It causes soreness, swelling, and redness at the tip of the penis. There are several possible sources for such irritation, including an infection such as genital herpes, a tight foreskin that is difficult to keep clean, or irritation caused by an allergic reaction to condoms or **spermicides (SPIR mih sydz)**.

Another form of balanitis, **balanitis xerotica obliterans (zah ROT ih kuh ob LIT eh ranz)**, has no known cause, and differs from the other forms in that the tip of the penis becomes pale and shrivelled instead of red and swollen, and the disorder can cause stricture of the urethral meatus.

The usual form of balanitis is treated by removing the cause and applying a soothing cream or ointment to relieve irritation. If infection is found, antibiotic cream may be necessary. If the foreskin is not retractable, it may have to be removed by circumcision **(SER kum SIZH un)**. In balanitis xerotica obliterans, the treatment may include surgical widening of the urethra.

Penile Warts

Penile warts are caused by the human papilloma virus. They can appear anywhere on the body, including the penis and the urethra. Since warts are an infection, they can be passed between sexual partners. Very small warts may need to be visualized via application of acetic acid and use of magnification. Penile warts can be treated with local application of podophyllin, a chemical that destroys the wart. Other treatments may include cryosurgery, which freezes wart tissue; electrosurgery, which destroys warts with electrical heat; and laser therapy, which "evaporates" wart tissue. Without treatment of both sexual partners, the warts could cause cell changes that may lead to cancer, especially of the cervix.

THE EFFECTS OF DIABETES MELLITUS ON EJACULATION

The man must be able to relax and contract the muscles that control erection and ejaculation in order to deliver sperm successfully into the vagina. Certain diseases and conditions can interfere with this process. Nerve damage due to diabetes mellitus can cause a condition in which semen is released back into the bladder instead of out through the urethra. This happens because the damaged nerves can no longer control the muscles that usually close the bladder entrance during sexual intercourse.

"Jock Itch"

Several different organisms or allergic reactions can cause rash and severe itching of the genitals. Some common causes are tinea and candidiasis, both of which are fungal infections. Such infections thrive in moist, dark, warm environments. Tight-fitting underwear or pants and friction on the skin can make these problems worse.

Treatment for jock itch includes use of an absorbent powder to dry the genital area, and use of soothing creams or liquids. Airing the genitals is also helpful, especially in very warm weather or tropical climates.

SEXUALLY TRANSMITTED DISEASES (STDs)

These diseases are passed from person to person through sexual contact. The public health department must be notified when these diseases are found because an effort is being made to eradicate them by finding and treating every affected person. A patient with one of these diseases must expect to be asked about sexual contacts, so that the person who passed the infection can be found and treated. Most of these diseases can be contracted only by sexual contact. Some individuals may be upset by questions about their sex lives, but the questions are required by law. Also, a person who has contracted an STD from a spouse or lover will have to deal with the question of how *that* person contracted the disease, which also may be difficult personally.

There are three reasons why STDs continue to be some of the world's most common diseases: (1) widespread unprotected sexual relations with multiple partners; (2) increased resistance of some organisms to antibiotics; and (3) delay in seeking treatment.

Gonorrhea

Gonorrhea is an infection caused by *Neisseria gonorrhoeae*, an organism we described earlier. The first site of infection is usually the genitals or urethra. There may be no outward signs or symptoms of the disease in some cases. However, in most cases the patient will have a spontaneous cloudy discharge, severe pain on urination, penile itching, and redness at the urinary meatus. If this goes untreated, large quantities of pus will appear. Prostatitis frequently develops, stricture in the male urethra or vas deferens can develop, and sterility can result. Gonorrhea can spread through the bloodstream and invade other body tissues, especially joints, bones, skin, and tendons.

The disease can be diagnosed by laboratory tests of pus to detect gonococci. Gonorrhea is usually treated with antibiotic drugs such as penicillin, but early detection is essential. The patient should not have sexual intercourse until the disease is eliminated to avoid passing it to the sexual partner. The partner should be tested for the disease as well.

Syphilis

Like gonorrhea, syphilis (**SIF ih liss**) is a bacterial infection that can be contracted due to sexual contact or intimate contact with an infectious lesion. It is caused by bacteria called *Treponema pallidum*. Syphilis has three stages.

The *first stage* causes small, painless sores called chancres (**SHANG kerz**) in the genital area. They are red, solid, and protruding. The chancres heal in a few weeks, but leave a scar. The bacteria circulate in the bloodstream while the chancres appear on the skin.

The *second stage* occurs about 6 weeks later. It causes a general infection, with fever, headache, swollen glands, a small, red, nonitching rash, and gray patches on the mucous membranes of the mouth.

The *third stage* of syphilis is delayed for several years, but once underway it can last for many years. It can cause loss of equilibrium, paralysis, insanity, or blindness, and can also affect the cardiovascular system severely.

Syphilis is diagnosed by the Venereal Disease Research Laboratory (VDRL) test and the rapid plasma reagin (RPR) test. Treatment with penicillin is successful except during the third phase. If the disease has progressed beyond the first two stages, or if it has begun to damage the brain during the second stage, it is not curable. Therefore, early treatment is very important. Also, the chancres are highly contagious. Anyone who has had sexual contact with the patient should also be tested and treated as soon as possible.

Genital Herpes

Genital herpes (**HUR peez**) is an infection of the skin in the genital area. There are two types of the causative virus: type I, the **herpes simplex virus**, which causes "fever blisters" or "cold sores," and type II, which involves the mucous membranes of the genital tract. Genital herpes can be spread by sexual contact with someone who has the disease or by contact with contaminated hands. Thus, a patient who has cold sores can infect his or her own genital area by touching the sores and then touching the genitals.

Genital herpes first causes severe pain, tenderness, itching, and fever. Blisters then appear on the skin of the vulva and sometimes also the thighs and buttocks. The blisters break and form painful ulcers, which may last for several weeks.

The disease is spread when blisters or ulcers are present. After the skin problems clear, the virus remains dormant in the body, and it may flare up again at any time. Active infection may be triggered by stress or for no apparent reason.

The most accurate diagnosis results from a positive virus culture on live tissue. The Tzanck smear test of ulcer fluid is also used.

There is no cure for genital herpes; antibiotics are not effective against viruses. Medical researchers are working to develop better preparations to ease the discomfort due to the blisters and ulcers. Use of condoms or diaphragms provides some protection from transmitting the virus during intercourse, but abstention from sexual contact while herpes is active is essential to prevent infecting the partner.

Chancroid

Chancroid (**SHANG kroyd**) produces an ulcer similar in appearance to a chancre. These ulcers appear on the genitals a few days after intercourse with an infected partner. They are painful and enlarge gradually. After a few weeks, the inguinal lymph nodes become swollen and tender, and the patient may have a fever, headache and a feeling of general illness.

This rare STD can be prevented by washing the genitals with soap and water after intercourse. It is diagnosed by the symptoms and by blood and urine tests. Chancroid can be treated easily with antibiotics, and further infection can be prevented by cleansing. If the foreskin becomes tightened over the tip of the penis, the foreskin may have to be slit or surgically removed (prepucectomy).

Chlamydial Infections

Chlamydial infections are among the most common STDs in the United States. Several strains of the organism are responsible for sexually transmitted genital and urinary infections in men and women. Diagnostic tests have been recently improved. The disease responds to certain antibiotics but not penicillin. The infection often exists with gonorrhea.

Lymphogranuloma Venereum

This rare STD is caused by a specific chlamydial organism. In **lymphogranuloma venereum (LIM foh GRAN yoo LOH mah veh NEE ree um)**, small, painless blisters form on the penis 1 month or more after exposure. The blisters quickly disappear and are followed by swelling of the inguinal lymph nodes, chills, fever, headache, joint pain, nausea, vomiting, and skin rashes. The lymph nodes form cavities that fill with fluid and drain into the lymphatic system.

Diagnosis is done by blood tests called complement fixation tests, which can detect a particular antibody in the blood. Treatment with selected antibiotics is usually completely successful. In a few cases, excess fluid in the lymph nodes must be removed with a needle (aspiration).

Acquired Immune Deficiency Syndrome (AIDS)

Acquired immune deficiency syndrome is increasingly a worldwide problem. (For a more thorough discussion of AIDS virus transmission, see the book on immunology in this series.) AIDS destroys the immune system during the advanced stage. It results from **human autoimmunodeficiency virus** (HIV) which infects the cells that protect the body against virus, bacteria, fungi, and parasites. When the body's immune system is weakened, many infections activate or reactivate to cause the common infections found in AIDS. Some low-grade infections that a healthy person can resist will cause diseases or infections in the presence of HIV.

HIV has three known routes of transmission: unprotected sexual contact through body fluids; shared blood or blood products; and from mother to fetus across the placental barrier or during birth or breast feeding. The virus will not penetrate the skin but enters through openings.

Within weeks of being infected with HIV, most people experience a brief illness (3 to 12 days) that appears to be flu, a cold, or mononucleosis. They complain of sore throat, fever, tender swollen lymph glands, body pains, rashes, or diarrhea. During the prolonged and variable time between early infection and the appearance of AIDS, (1 to 10 years), most people have no symptoms except swollen lymph nodes. They may experience the chickenpox virus in the form of shingles, herpes zoster, fever blisters, or tuberculosis. Recurrent yeast infections also may develop. There may be severe fatigue, fever or night sweats, diarrhea, and unexplained weight loss.

HIV can be diagnosed by the enzyme linked immunosorbent assay (ELISA) test.

False positive results may occur, and a positive result is confirmed by the more definitive Western blot assay. These tests will reveal HIV antibodies in the blood. A positive test indicates only that the patient has been exposed to HIV and may be capable of transmitting the disease; but does not necessarily mean that he or she will develop AIDS.

Diagnosis may also be made by detecting an opportunistic infection (an infection by an organism that causes disease only in a person whose resistance is lowered). The most common AIDS-defining infection is pneumonocytis (NOO moh SISS tiss) pneumonia. This is a slowly developing infection that occurs only in immunosuppressed patients. Kaposi's sarcoma (KAP oh seez sar COH muh), a rare red to purple skin tumor, may also be found.

Both diagnosis and treatment have become more difficult because several different strains of HIV have been identified and been proven to mutate (change). Although various approaches to treating AIDS are being studied, there is yet no cure. One antiviral drug, zidovudine (or AZT), has been shown to reduce the number of early deaths and repeated infections from opportunistic pathogens. Since the disease can affect any body system, symptomatic treatment is presently performed. Patients who have chosen to do so are sometimes given investigational drugs and then observed to determine the

drug's effectiveness.

Condom use during intercourse is strongly encouraged as a way to guard against being infected with AIDS, but the only certain way to avoid sexually transmitted HIV at this time is through abstinence or monogamous sexual activity with an uninfected partner.

Hepatitis B

Hepatitis B is transmitted sexually and by using contaminated needles or blood products. It is a viral hepatitis that causes acute liver inflammation; liver, muscle, and joint pain; lymph node enlargement; headache; loss of appetite; and nausea and vomiting. Fever may also occur. Later symptoms include weight loss, dark yellow urine, jaundice, liver inflammation, and tenderness.

There is no cure for the disease, and treatment is supportive. A vaccine is available to health care workers and other high-risk individuals. The vaccine has been recommended as part of the routine immunizations given to all newborns. A diagnosed individual should abstain from sexual intercourse until determined to be noninfectious. Six to 10 percent of infected individuals will become chronic carriers of the virus.

Pubic Lice

These lice are also called crabs. They cling to the pubic hair and are transmitted by sexual contact. They feed on blood, so they cannot survive in bedding or unused clothing. The lice themselves are visible with the unaided eye. They lay eggs that are quite small but can just barely be seen attached to the hairs in the pubic area, around the anus, and sometimes on the eyebrows or other body hair. The lice cause itching. If a patient has pubic (**PEW bick**) lice, he may have other STDs and should be tested for them. Sexual contacts should also be treated for the lice and tested for other problems.

ABNORMAL GROWTHS

Cysts of the Epididymis

Especially in a man over age 40, cysts or fluid-filled sacs often form on the epididymis. They may grow large enough to be noticeable, but they rarely cause symptoms or even damage. A painless swelling in the area of the testes should be examined by a biopsy to detect malignancy. However, if the swelling is caused by a cyst, it usually needs no further treatment. In a few cases, the cyst becomes large enough to cause discomfort, and must be removed. The surgery may reduce sperm production in the affected testis.

Hydrocele

Hydrocele (HY droh seel) is a condition that looks like a growth. The sheath around each testis normally is lubricated with fluid to allow the gland to move within the scrotum. Sometimes this fluid accumulates in abnormal amounts, causing a soft, painless swelling around the testis. Once hydrocele begins, very often the fluid continues to accumulate and the problem recurs even after treatment. Treatment consists of removing excess fluid periodically to reduce the swelling. Surgical removal of the fluid and sheath around the testis is curative. This is called **hydrocelectomy (HY droh see LECK toh mee)**.

Varicocele

Varicocele (VAR ih koh SEEL) also causes swelling around the testes, but for a different reason. In this disorder, the veins that carry blood away from the gland constrict. This causes a mild pain, especially after exercise or in hot weather. The condition is not serious, but may decrease the sperm count, resutling in infertility. It can be treated by having the patient wear an athletic supporter or tight underwear. In severe cases, the affected veins can be removed.

Benign Enlargement of the Prostate

This condition, **benign prostatic hypertrophy (hy PER troh fee)** occurs to some extent in almost every man over age 45 or 50. As part of the aging process, extra deposits of normal prostate tissue grow on the gland, making it larger. The texture of the gland may change as well, making it stiff or even rigid. In many cases, neither of these changes causes problems. In severe cases, however, constriction of the urethra may occur.

The symptoms of severe prostatic enlargement are weak urine flow combined with the frequent urge to urinate. There may also be hematuria. Obstruction of the urinary tract may also cause bladder and kidney infections, with accompanying symptoms. In a few cases, the urethra is completely blocked and the bladder fills with urine, until the abdomen swells.

Diagnosis of an enlarged prostate is made by palpating the organ through the rectum and examining the urinary tract to detect obstruction and infection. Intravenous pyelography and cystography commonly are used to identify any obstruction and its effects on urine flow. Ultrasound scan of the lower abdomen will reveal the size of the prostate. If the gland has become rigid, a needle biopsy may be necessary to determine whether a malignant growth is present.

Treatment begins with relieving urinary retention, by catheter if necessary, and eliminating infection in the prostate gland and the urinary tract. If the obstruction of the urethra is not severe, the physician may simply advise the patient to avoid drinking large amounts of fluid (especially alcohol, which has a diuretic effect), to urinate whenever he has the urge, and to be alert for symptoms of recurring infection. In more severe cases, surgical removal of the abnormal growth may be necessary. There are several techniques available for this, but transurethral resection is the most common.

CANCERS OF THE MALE REPRODUCTIVE SYSTEM

Cancer of the Prostate

Prostate cancer is quite common in men over age 60. It is slow-growing and commonly causes no symptoms for many years. For this reason, it often is not discovered until it has metastasized to the lymph nodes near the prostate or to the pelvic bone. Although enlarged prostate does not appear to cause prostate cancer, the two conditions frequently occur together. In fact, a malignancy may be discovered by coincidence when apparently benign extra tissue is removed from the gland and tested.

Symptoms of prostate cancer are usually those of urinary tract infection, possibly including hematuria. The cancer can be detected by palpating the prostate gland. If it feels hard or has hard areas, the physician will suspect a malignancy. If the cancer has spread to the bones and lymph nodes without causing urinary tract symptoms, the first symptoms may be pain in the lower spine and weight loss.

Prostate cancer is diagnosed by a biopsy of the gland and examination of the tissue. The tissue may be removed by transurethral resection or by aspiration (needle biopsy). A blood test for prostatic-specific antigen (PSA) also is done to detect this antigen, which rises in patients with prostate cancer and other prostate disorders. This relatively new test allows earlier detection of prostate cancer than was formerly possible. Additional tests may include bone scans, computed tomography, intravenous pyelography, and transrectal ultrasonography. The latter test may be performed in the physician's office or radiology department, along with the prostate biopsy.

Treatment of prostate cancer that is discovered early usually involves removal of the gland and surrounding tissues, followed by radiation therapy. In a patient who will probably die of other causes before the cancer spreads, the physician may recommend relief of symptoms, also known as **palliation (pall ee AY shun)**, instead.

Treatment for prostate cancer generally depends on the stage of the cancer. In stage A, the tumor is in the prostate only, is not palpable, and causes no symptoms. This type of tumor may require surgery, radiation, or simply close follow-up. In stage B, the tumor affects only the prostate, is palpable, and typically produces no symptoms. It usually requires surgery or radiation. In stage C, the tumor affects the prostate and nearby areas, and may cause difficulty with urination. This type of tumor may be treated with surgery, radiation, or both. It also may require hormone therapy to decrease testosterone production and block the activity of other male hormones. In stage D, the tumor spreads to the bones and other parts of the body, producing such problems as bone pain, weight loss, and fatigue. For this type of tumor, treatment usually includes hormones and chemotherapy.

Decisions about the best type of treatment for this disease also depend on other factors. These include the patient's age and general health, the stage of the cancer when it is discovered, and the patient's preferences. Cure rates are as high as 60 to 70 percent for some stages of prostate cancer. In late stages, the cure rate is much lower.

Cancer of the Testis

Cancer of the testis occurs most often in men between age 25 and 35. An undescended testis is especially susceptible to cancer, for no known reason. The condition is almost always painless. The only symptom may be swelling or enlargement of the affected testis, which the patient may not notice until it becomes quite large and heavy. Hydrocele fluid retention (in the scrotum) may accompany the tumor. One type of testicular tumor secretes hormones that may cause breast swelling. This type is the most difficult to cure.

Cancer of the testis metastasizes fairly quickly. It may begin as a painless lump in the testis, gradually involve the entire testis and epididymis, and then spread to the lymph nodes in the lower abdomen. From there, the cancer may spread to the liver or lungs.

Preliminary diagnosis of cancer of the testis is made by palpating the testis. If hydrocele is present, the excess fluid may have to be drained before the physician can properly feel the shape and texture of a swelling of the testis. Blood tests, x-ray studies, ultrasound scans, and other tests are usually done to determine what type of tumor is present, what stage it has reached, and whether it has metastasized. These are all factors that help determine the best treatment for the cancer.

Depending on the results of these tests, the treatment may include radiation, surgery, and/or chemotherapy. In most cases, the affected testis must be removed surgically in an orchiectomy. Usually, the disease affects only one testicle, so most patients are fertile (able to have children) and potent (able to have erections) after the operation. The patient's chances of survival depend on the type of tumor and how quickly it was discovered and treated. With some tumors, survival rates are higher than 95 percent. New discoveries about the use of chemo-

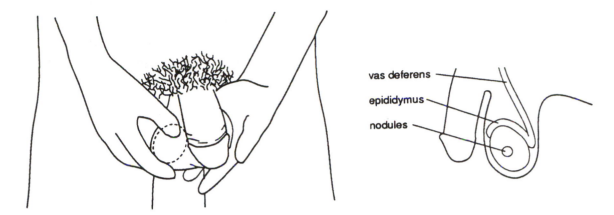

Figure 19: Self-examination for testicular cancer.

therapy are mainly responsible for improved treatment success.

Medical experts encourage men between ages 20 and 34 to examine their testicles each month for early detection of cancer (see Figure 19). Since prognosis is good if testicular cancer is detected early, this 3-minute examination may play a significant role in early detection.

To perform a testicular self-examination, the patient is instructed to:

1. Select any day of the month and perform the examination on that day each month.
2. Examine the scrotum after a warm bath or shower when the scrotal skin is most relaxed.
3. Support the scrotum with one hand and examine each testicle separately by rolling it gently between the thumb and fingers. Check for hard lumps or knots. This should NOT be painful.
4. Contact the physician if any changes or abnormalities are noted.

Cancer of the Penis

This type of cancer is rare, and extremely rare in circumcised men. It occurs as a sore, ulcer, or lump on the foreskin or the glans penis beneath the foreskin. The foreskin may become too tight to retract, and an infection may occur in the same area. The cancer usually spreads first to the shaft of the penis, then to the lymph nodes in the groin. There, it will cause swelling and sometimes tenderness or pain if an infection is present. If the cancer spreads beyond the lymph nodes in the groin, the patient's chances of survival are poor.

Diagnosis of cancer of the penis is made by a biopsy of the growth and by blood tests. The growth may resemble syphilis, chancroid, or penile warts, so these possibilities are investigated. Once a diagnosis of cancer is made, treatment depends on whether or not the cancer has spread. If it has not spread, the foreskin and tumor can be removed. Some physicians use radiation therapy rather than surgery to remove the tumor. Later stages of the disease may require amputation of the end of the penis, and possibly removal or radiation of the affected lymph glands.

STRUCTURAL PROBLEMS

The structure of the male reproductive system may be abnormal because of a genetic or other congenital problem. Injury from persistent infection or from trauma can also cause structural problems.

Hypospadias and Epispadias

These conditions are congenital, and probably hereditary, abnormalities of the penis and urethra. **Chordee (KOR dee),** or abnormal curvature of the penis, can occur with either of the two. **Hypospadias (HY poh SPAY dee as)** is a combination of abnormalities including ventral (toward the front) chordee, misplacement of the urinary meatus on the ventral side of the penis, an abnormally small penis, and sometimes the presence of a partial or complete vagina and uterus in a child with a male chromosome pattern. Occasionally, ventral chordee occurs alone, without any other abnormalities. **Epispadias (EP ih SPAY dee as)** is an abnormality in which the urinary meatus is on the dorsal, or back, side of the penis. It often includes dorsal chordee. Any of these problems may involve some degree of urinary tract obstruction.

In most cases, these conditions can be corrected surgically in childhood, usually before the child enters school. The goals of surgery are to correct any urinary blockage and to make normal sexual activity possible.

Cryptorchidism (Undescended Testes)

Some boys are born with one or both testes still in the abdominal cavity rather than in the scrotum. In the embryo, the testes are formed near the kidneys, and normally descend into the scrotum in the last few weeks before birth. The undescended organ may descend on its own, in the first 2 years of life or at puberty. However, the ability of the affected testis to produce sperm may be reduced because of a congenital abnormality in the testis or because the higher temperature inside the abdomen can damage sperm-producing cells. Cryptorchidism may be accompanied by an inguinal hernia.

Often the only symptom of the problem is the absence of the testis in the scrotum.

The scrotum may atrophy, or shrink, on that side. Sometimes the doctor can feel the undescended testis in the groin. Treatment usually is delayed until the child is about age 5, to give the testis an opportunity to descend naturally. If it does not, the child is given hormones by mouth or injection, to try to stimulate descent of the testis. If this is ineffective, an operation called **orchiopexy (OR kee oh PECK see)** is done to move the testis into the proper position. The surgeon must be careful to keep the blood vessels attached to the testis intact. Otherwise, the testis may die from lack of circulation. If a hernia is found, the surgeon will repair it during the operation. In some cases, the undescended testis must be removed, because it is abnormal or damaged. This is done to prevent later development of cancer of the testis.

In many cases, fertility is reduced, but only one testis is affected, so the boy will be able to produce children. When both testes are undescended, the patient may be infertile. However, impotence rarely occurs, because the damaged testes continue to produce testosterone even if they do not produce sperm.

FUNCTIONAL PROBLEMS

Torsion of the Testis

Torsion, or twisting, of the testis is most common in young men and boys, but it can happen in infants and older men. It is especially common in males with undescended testes. The testis is suspended in the scrotum and held by the spermatic cord. Sometimes, because of an abnormality in the structures around the testis, or an abnormal movement, or for no apparent reason, the spermatic cord becomes twisted. This reduces or even blocks the blood supply to the testis, causing pain, swelling, inflammation, and cell death.

In some cases, the testis untwists by itself, but it usually remains twisted until it is manually or surgically replaced into its proper position.

The symptoms of torsion are pain, redness, and swelling in the scrotum, and sometimes, in severe cases, nausea and vomiting. Diagnosis may be difficult, especially in an older patient, because the symptoms are similar to those of epididymitis. Immediate treatment of torsion is essential to prevent damage to the testis. Therefore, surgery may be done even if the diagnosis is not certain. A combination of an ultrasound scan and the use of an instrument called a Doppler stethoscope can often confirm the diagnosis.

In some cases, the physician can untwist the testis without opening the scrotum. However, torsion tends to recur, so even in cases where it untwists without treatment, surgery is advised. In the operation, the surgeon untwists the spermatic cord and stitches the testis into its proper place with permanent sutures to prevent recurrence. If the spermatic cord remains twisted for more than 48 hours, the testis probably will be removed, because it will be too badly damaged to function, and the dead cells may harbor gangrene.

Impotence

Impotence (IM poh tenss) means inability to either achieve or maintain an erection. This condition prevents sexual activity in the male. Impotence can be caused by psychological problems, physical problems, or a combination of the two. It is sometimes difficult to distinguish one from the other, yet the cause must be identified before the problem can be treated successfully. Some of the possible physical causes of impotence are drugs, especially those prescribed for hypertension or depression; chronic alcoholism with liver damage; hormone imbalance; diabetes; nerve damage; and circulation problems. Possible psychological causes include severe depression, marital conflict, and abnormal stress.

Diagnosis and treatment of impotence are approached at first by extensive interviewing of the patient and careful review of his medical history. A personal or familial history of diabetes mellitus, treatment for high blood pressure, or a history of alcoholism are possible clues. If the cause is purely physical, the patient will not have spontaneous erections at night and will not be able to stimulate an erection by masturbation, so these factors must be explored. Blood tests to measure hormone levels, and other tests of nervous system and cardiovascular system function may be useful. An evaluation of drugs (prescription and nonprescription) that the patient is taking may help identify the source of the problem.

Treatment for impotence depends on the findings from the tests and interviews. Some experts estimate that impotence has a physical cause in about 10 percent of cases. Some of these problems can be treated by adjustments in medication or by correction of hormone imbalances. In some instances, a penile implant of a semiflexible rod or a fluid-filled prosthesis has proved satisfactory. But some physical causes cannot be corrected, and lead to permanent impairment of sexual activity. If no physical problems can be identified, the patient and possibly his spouse or sexual partner will be referred to a sex therapist or psychiatrist.

Several other treatments may be helpful for a patient with impotence. Two types of penile implants can be surgically implanted to allow the patient to have an erection. The semirigid rod creates a permanent erection, but is flexible enough to be bent toward the body for easy concealment. The inflatable prothesis contains a pump, reservoir, and release valve, and lets the patient control his erections as desired. Self-injection of papaverine into the spongy erectile tissue of the penis may allow temporary erection for some patients.

Priapism

Priapism (PRY ah pizm) is an erection that persists in the absence of sexual stimulation and will not relax. This condition is rare, but it is extremely serious. It can cause impotence due to permanent damage to the tissues in the penis. It occurs because, for some reason, blood that enters the penis is prevented from flowing out again. Initial treatment includes ice water enemas and removal of excess blood from the penis with a needle. The penis may also be irrigated with phenylephrine (Neo-Synephrine) solution. An anticoagulant drug may then be injected into the penis to prevent clots from forming and blocking the circulation again. If these measures are ineffective, immediate surgery is required to remove blockages in the blood vessels and restore normal circulation.

Peyronie's Disease

This disease occurs almost exclusively in men over age 45. The layer of tissue that covers the corpora cavernosa of the penis becomes fibrous and sometimes accumulates calcium deposits or even ossifies (hardens like bone). During erection, the penis bends in the direction of the fibrous deposits instead of being straight. The problem may cause pain, especially at first. If the penis is bent far enough, sexual intercourse becomes impossible.

Some of the possible approaches to treatment for **Peyronie's (pay RON eez) disease** include low-dose radiation and attempts to remove the deposits surgically. No single treatment has produced reliable results for this disorder, and it may not be correctable in some cases.

Phimosis

Phimosis (fy MOH siss) is tightening of the foreskin in an uncircumcised male. The foreskin cannot be retracted, usually because of an infection that has developed under it. The infection may be caused by accumulated debris. The problem can usually be prevented by careful and regular cleaning under the foreskin.

The major symptom of phimosis is inability to retract the foreskin. It usually is accompanied by redness, swelling, pain, and sometimes pus around the tip of the penis. Treatment typically requires that the foreskin be slit to relieve pressure and provide access to the infection. Antibiotics and soaking are prescribed to reduce inflammation. Circumcision is then done to prevent the problem from recurring.

Hemospermia

This term means blood in the semen. The condition is not serious. It usually is caused by the rupture of small blood vessels in the urethra which occurs during ejaculation. The blood vessels repair themselves quickly, without treatment. The only danger in **hemospermia (HEE moh SPER mee ah)** is that the blood may originate in the urinary tract. If it does, it may indicate a serious condition, such as kidney or bladder cancer, a severe urinary tract infection, or urinary retention. These disorders all require immediate treatment.

Fill in the blanks.

1. Three instruments or techniques used specifically for male reproductive problems are:

   a. _____

   b. _____

   c. _____

2. A transurethral resection is done with a _____ .

3. Prostatitis is most common in _____ .

4. Give three symptoms of acute prostatitis.

   a. _____

   b. _____

   c. _____

5. _____ sometimes occurs as a side effect of prostatectomy.

6. Chlamydial or bacterial infections or trauma (injury) can cause _____ .

7. Inflammation of the testes, sometimes caused by mumps, is called _____ .

8. Two disorders of the male reproductive system that cause swelling and fluid accumulation are _____ and _____ .

9. Constriction of blood vessels can cause two disorders of the male reproductive system:_____ and _____ .

10. Two instruments that are used to treat benign enlargement of the prostate are the _____ and _____ .

11. The rarest form of cancer of the male reproductive system is _____ .

12. Abnormal downward curvature of the penis is called _____ .

13. Three disorders of the reproductive system that most often affect older men are:

    a. _____

    b. _____

    c. _____

14. Cryptorchidism is a _____ condition that is corrected by a surgical procedure called _____ .

15. Three possible causes of impotence are:

    a. _____

    b. _____

    c. _____

(continued next page)

True or False.

16. _____ Penicillin is one treatment for prostatitis.

17. _____ Diseases of the male reproductive system that may be treated with antibiotics include prostatitis, epididymitis, balanitis, chancroid, and lymphogranuloma venereum.

Short answers.

18. Prostatic-specific antigen is a blood test used to diagnose_____ .

19. Name three sexually transmitted diseases (STDs).

    a. _____

    b. _____

    c. _____

20. Give three reasons why STDs are so difficult to control.

    a. _____

    b. _____

    c. _____

21. List five ways to reduce the transmission of STDs:

    a. _____

    b. _____

    c. _____

    d. _____

    e. _____

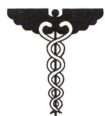

Knowledge Objectives

After completing this chapter, you should be able to:

- name the internal female reproductive organs
- identify the location and function of the uterine tubes
- describe the structure of the uterus
- locate and describe the vagina and list its three main functions
- name and describe the external female reproductive organs
- describe the structures of the breast
- identify the four hormones that most affect the menstrual cycle and where they are made
- describe the events of the menstrual cycle, including those in the menstrual, follicular, and luteal phases
- define menarche and menopause

The Female Reproductive System

INTRODUCTION

The next two chapters deal with the anatomy, physiology, and diseases of the female reproductive organs which are different from those of the male. Because the **embryo, fetus,** and newborn are so closely linked to the mother in pregnancy and delivery, these stages of development will be covered in Chapter 7. The brief discussion of pediatrics (treatment of children) will focus on those aspects that might be treated, or at least diagnosed, during or soon after delivery.

The medical specialties that diagnose and treat the systems and diseases described in these chapters include:

- **gynecologists (GY nuh KOL oh jist),** specialists who deal with the physiology and diseases of the female reproductive organs, including endocrinology and reproduction
- **obstetricians (OB steh TRISH un),** who specialize in the care of women during pregnancy, labor, delivery, and postpartum recovery
- **obstetrician/gynecologists,** who specialize in a combination of the two

- **neonatologists (NEE oh nay TAHL oh jist),** specialists who may consult with mothers just before delivery, but who are involved primarily in care of newborns having a wide variety of disorders
- **pediatricians (PEE dee ah TRISH un),** who specialize in the development, care, and diseases of infants and children
- **family practice physicians,** who treat both parents and children
- **general practitioners**, who may provide any or all of the services above.

The female reproductive system establishes, protects, gives birth to, and nourishes new life, thus maintaining the human species. As part of this process, the **ovaries (OH vah reez)** produce **ova (OH vah)** (singular, ovum) or eggs. This is the female's contribution to conception. The male sperm provides the additional genetic material needed to start the development of an embyro. Some parts of the genital system provide sexual stimulation and pleasure, which in turn prepare other parts of the body for intercourse and sperm deposit through lubrication and other mechanisms.

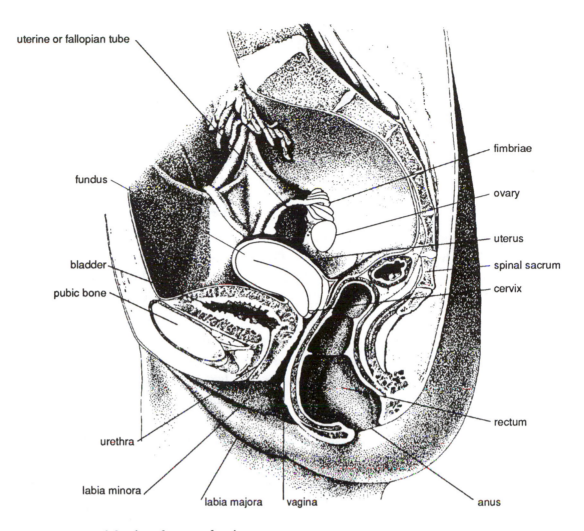

Labels on figure:
- uterine or fallopian tube
- fundus
- bladder
- pubic bone
- urethra
- labia minora
- labia majora
- vagina
- fimbriae
- ovary
- uterus
- spinal sacrum
- cervix
- rectum
- anus

Figure 20: Sagittal section of the female reproductive organs.

STRUCTURES AND ORGANS

There are internal and external structures and organs of the female reproductive system. The internal parts include two ovaries, two **uterine (YOO ter in)** or **fallopian (fah LOH pee an) tubes**, a **uterus (YOO ter us)**, and a **vagina (vah JY nah)** (see Figure 20). The external structures include the **vulva (VUL vah)** (see Figure 23) and the **breasts** (see Figure 24). The bones of the pelvis also play an important part in the structure of the reproductive system. The functioning of the system is governed in part by hormones secreted by the pituitary gland located at the base of the brain.

The location and general function of each of these elements of the reproductive system will be described first. To help you understand how the system works and what can go wrong with it, a series of overlapping cycles of chemical and physical changes will be described next, and will include the changes that occur during the **menstrual (MEN stroo al) cycle** and **pregnancy**.

DEVELOPMENT AND CHANGE

The female reproductive organs are designed for change and adaptation. Throughout childhood before puberty (sexual maturity), reproductive organs are inactive. During this time, a region within the hypothalamus of the brain slowly matures. When the region has matured, the hypothalamus secretes a hormone called gonadotropin-releasing hormone (GnRH). The pituitary gland starts to make and store follicle-stimulating hormone (FSH), which causes development of egg sacs within the ovaries.

These events usually occur between ages 11 and 14. Secondary sexual characteristics also appear at this time: the breasts develop; fat is deposited beneath the skin, particularly in the hips and breasts; the pelvis widens and lightens; and hair grows in the pubic area and under the arms. At about the same time, the menstrual cycle begins. The menstrual cycle continues and causes changes in the reproductive tract every month for the next 30 to 50 years.

If pregnancy occurs, the system undergoes more dramatic changes. A new life develops within the system, changing the shape and position of the organs and calling on all their resources and resiliency to complete the process that ends in childbirth. Following childbirth, the organs gradually return to almost the same shape and position as before, and the cycle continues.

At the end of the childbearing years, the menstrual cycle gradually comes to an end with **menopause (MEN oh pawz).** The organs of the reproductive system again adapt to change. They gradually atrophy, or shrink.

BASIC FEMALE ANATOMY

An understanding of basic female anatomy begins with an idea of how the reproductive organs are situated in relation to the rest of the body (see Figure 20). The organs include the ovaries, uterine tubes, uterus, **cervix (SIR vicks),** and vagina. They are located in the pelvis, between the rectum, which is the inferior end of the digestive tract, and the urinary bladder and urethra, which are part of the urinary tract. The rectum curves between the spine and the uterus and vagina. The uterus is usually tilted forward, and the urinary bladder is located inferior to it and anterior to the vagina (see Figure 20).

PELVIC GIRDLE

The pelvic **(PEL vick)** girdle (see Figure 21) surrounds all of these organs and joins with the spine posteriorly, behind the rectum. The pelvic bones are fused to form a circular framework near the base of the spine with an opening in the middle. The hip bones form the sides of the circle, and the pubic bone forms the front. The pelvis is joined to the sacral section of the spine posteriorly, at the sacroiliac joint. The coccyx, which is made up of the last five bones of the spine, protrudes slightly inferior to the pelvic opening. The hip joints are attached to the outside edges of the hip bones. The reproductive organs, rectum, urinary bladder, and urethra are inside the pelvic cavity, protected from injury by its bony structure.

The female pelvis differs from the male pelvis in two major ways: first, because the female pelvic girdle houses several reproductive organs, it is wider and has fewer bony projections. The diameter of the opening is larger in the female, and projections on the surrounding bones are smaller or tilted differently so that they will not interfere with passage of the fetus through the birth canal. Second, the opening at the center of the female pelvic girdle is circular. The male pelvis, on the other hand, is narrowed at the front. If you could look down on a male and a female pelvis from above, you would see that the male pelvis has a heart-shaped opening, while the female pelvis has a

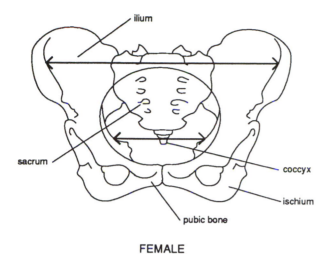

ilium

sacrum

coccyx

ischium

pubic bone

FEMALE

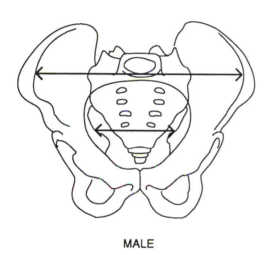

MALE

Figure 21: Comparison of the male and female pelvis.

rounded opening (see Figure 21).

Two main reasons explain these differences: first, most of the male reproductive organs, with the exception of the prostate and vesicles, are outside the pelvic cavity; and second, the male pelvis does not have to accommodate the fetus.

The structures outside the vaginal opening are called the external reproductive organs, external genitals, or the vulva. These organs are located between the pubic bone and the anus. They are critical parts of the system and are most susceptible to infection because of their location on the surface of the body.

The breasts are anchored to the front of the chest between the second and sixth ribs. They are considered part of the reproductive system and are a distinctive characteristic of female anatomy.

INTERNAL REPRODUCTIVE ORGANS

Ovaries

The two ovaries are similar in shape to almonds and are about the size of walnuts (see Figure 20). They are located on either side of the uterus, approximately even with the top of the uterus or slightly above it. Each ovary is attached to a broad ligament, which also holds that side of the uterus in its place in the pelvic cavity. The ovaries are also attached to the uterus by the ovarian ligaments, but they are not actually attached to the uterine tubes.

The ovaries are glands that contain egg germs called **oogonia (OH oh GOH nee ah)** (sing., **OH oh GON ee um**), each encased in its own sac called a **follicle** or ovarian follicle. Women are born with a finite number of ovarian follicles at birth, approximately 400,000. After puberty, the follicles begin to ripen, a few at a time. Usually each ovary produces a mature ovum every other month from puberty until menopause, except during pregnancy. This process is called **oogenesis (OH oh JEN eh siss)**. The release of the egg is called **ovulation (OH vew LAY shun)**. The egg supply diminishes naturally over time. When the supply of eggs is exhausted, the woman has reached menopause. The eggs are used up whether they are fertilized or not. Birth control pills neither cause the eggs to be stored nor accelerate their loss.

Both oogenesis and ovulation will be discussed further in Chapter 7. The ovaries also secrete the hormones **estrogen (ES troh jen)** and **progesterone (proh JEST teh rohn)** as part of the menstrual cycle.

The center of each ovary is called the medulla. It is made up of connective tissue and contains blood vessels that nourish the entire structure. The outside, or cortex, of the ovary is made up of a thin outer layer of germinal epithelial cells and an inner layer of ovarian follicles.

Uterine Tubes

The uterine tubes, sometimes called fallopian tubes or oviducts, are the ducts through which the ripened ova travel from the ovary to the uterus. Closest to the ovary, the uterine tube widens and its funnel-shaped opening has finger-like projections called **fimbriae (FIM bree ee)** (see Figure 22). The fimbriae sweep across the outside of the ovary and pick up the egg as it emerges from the ovary. Tubal infections can damage the delicate fimbriae causing fertility problems.

Since the ovary and uterine tube are not connected, an ovum occasionally escapes into the pelvic cavity instead of going into the tube. The uterine tubes curl around the top of the ovary with the fimbriae at one end and connect to the top edge of the uterus at the other (see Figure 22).

Fertilization of an ovum by a sperm usually occurs in the outer third of the uterine tube, closest to the ovary. Whether it is fertilized or not, the ovum normally continues down the tube and into the uterus. Each tube is about 10 cm long, and is made up of three layers of tissue. The inner layer consists of mucous membrane with tiny, hairlike filaments called **cilia (SIL ee ah)** along its walls. The middle layer is composed of smooth muscle, and the outer layer is made up of the same kind of tissue as the **peritoneum**, the lining of the inner cavities. Because the uterine tubes connect to the uterus and thus to the vagina, they can become infected in the same way as those organs. The ovaries are far less susceptible to infection from the outside because they are not actually connected to the uterine tubes.

Uterus

Above the cervix is the uterus, a pear-shaped organ that holds and nourishes the developing embryo and fetus (see Figure 20). In a woman who has never been pregnant, the uterus is approximately 7 cm high, 5 cm wide at the top (the widest part), and 3 cm thick and weighs 2 ounces. The uterus and cervix lie at right angles to the vagina, and the body of the uterus is tilted slightly forward. It is anchored in place by eight ligaments (two broad ligaments, two uterosacral ligaments, posterior and anterior ligaments, and two round ligaments). All of these ligaments are flexible, to allow for fetal growth and uterine expansion in pregnancy. The uterine walls are elastic and strong. This is necessary because labor and childbirth involve powerful contractions that move the fetus down the birth canal (vagina) and out of the mother's body.

The inner wall of the uterus, called the **endometrium (en doh MEE tree um)** anchors and nourishes the fertilized egg (see

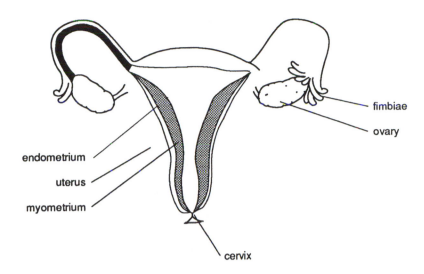

Figure 22: Relationship of ovaries, uterine or fallopian tubes, and uterus, anterior view.

Figure 22). It has three layers. The superficial layer is made of epithelial cells. It builds up and is shed as part of the menstrual cycle, or it receives the fertilized egg, which implants itself where endometrial blood vessels and glands supply nourishment during pregnancy. The middle layer is made up of spongy tissue, and is also shed each month except in pregnancy. The deep layer, which is permanent, is full of spiral-shaped blood vessels called arterioles, which supply blood to the superficial layer. It holds the endometrium to the muscular layer beneath.

Surrounding the endometrium is a muscular wall called the **myometrium (my oh MEET ree um)** (see Figure 22), which is made up of three types of muscle. The first type are longitudinal muscle fibers that contract to help expel the fetus. The second type are fibers that encircle large blood vessels and close them off when the placenta separates. The third type are fibers that surround the end of the uterine tubes and the cervical os to prevent reflux of menstrual blood. The outside of the uterus, like the outside of the uterine tubes, is made up of peritoneal tissue.

The top of the uterus is called the **fundus (FUN dus).** The upper part, including the fundus, is the body of the uterus. The uterus is widest at the fundus which is thicker and more rounded than the other uterine walls, bulging at the top. The uterine tubes enter the uterus just beneath the fundus.

Cervix

At the opposite end, the uterus narrows into a section called the cervix (see Figure 22). The cervix opens into the vagina. Normally, the cervix secretes an alkaline mucus that protects the sperm from the acidity of vaginal secretions. Sperm can live in this mucus for up to 3 days. Small sacs lining the cervix called crypts produce the mucus. These sacs also hold sperm and can continue to release the sperm upward toward the uterine cavity for several hours after intercourse. The thickness and amount of cervical mucus vary during the menstrual cycle. The quality of the mucus at the time of ovulation can help a physician determine a woman's degree of fertility.

Vagina

The vagina is a muscular tube that leads from the uterus to the outside (see Figure 20). It is located between the rectum, which is posterior to it, and the urethra and bladder, which are anterior to it. The structure is normally 7 to 8 cm long and is very expandable. It is tilted back from its outside opening to the cervix. In a young woman who has not had sexual intercourse, the outer opening of the vagina is usually surrounded and partially covered by a membrane called the **hymen (HY men)**. This membrane is broken by intercourse, or sometimes by strenuous exercise. If the hymen covers the entire opening, it must be opened surgically at puberty to allow the normal passage of menstrual flow.

The vagina has three major functions: it is the lower end of the birth canal, it receives the male organ and sperm during intercourse, and it provides a passageway to the outside for menstrual flow and other secretions from the reproductive system.

EXTERNAL REPRODUCTIVE ORGANS

Vulva

The external female genitals are collectively called the vulva (see Figure 23) and include the outer lips (**labia majora; LAY bee ah mah JOR ah)**, the inner lips (**labia minora; LAY bee ah mih NOR ah)**, and the **clitoris (KLIT oh ris)**.

Above the vulva body is a pad of fatty tissue over the pubic bone that is covered with coarse pubic hairs. This area is called the **mons pubis (MONZ PEW biss)**. The labia majora, also called the vulval lips, extend almost to the anus. The labia majora is a fold of skin that covers the other vulval organs and protects them. The labia majora has hair on the outside and is smooth on the inside. It is composed of glands and fat.

Inside this protective layer is a second, similar fold of skin called the labia minora, which provides further padding and protection. The labia minora is a modified form of skin tissue. It closes along the midline of the vulva. The area inside the two labia is called the **vestibule (VES tih byool)**.

Just inside the vulval lips in the front is the clitoris , a small structure made of erectile tissue similar to the penis in the male. It is covered by the **prepuce (PREE pyooss)**, which is a fold of skin similar to the foreskin or prepuce in the male, but much smaller. The clitoris becomes erect in a woman who is sexually stimulated, as part of **orgasm**, the sexual climax.

Urethral Opening

The next structure, moving from front to back, is the urethral opening called the urinary meatus. Urine flows from the urinary bladder, through the urethra, and then outside the body through the opening.

Vaginal Orifice

Behind the urethral opening is the vaginal

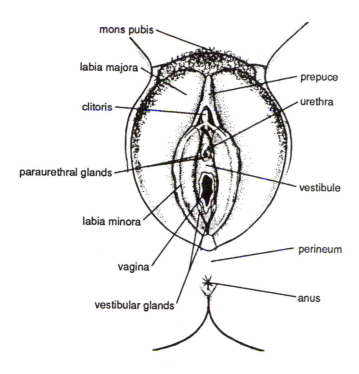

Figure 23: Female external genitalia.

orifice. Between the two openings are the two ducts of the **paraurethral (PAR ah yoo REE thruhl)** glands. On either side of the vaginal orifice, the ducts from vestibular glands emerge, one on each side. These glands secrete mucus that lubricates the vagina before and after intercourse. Both pairs are susceptible to infection, particularly in cases of gonorrhea.

Perineum
Behind the vulva is the **anus (AY nus)** (see Figure 23), the passage from the rectum to the outside. Between the anus and the external genitals is an area of muscle called the **perineum (PER ih NEE um)**. This muscle provides support for the internal organs of the pelvic cavity, and it is under a great deal of stress during childbirth. Sometimes it tears during labor, and it is difficult to repair because such tears may be irregular and deep.

To make delivery easier, some physicians will make a surgical cut in the perineum during the process of delivery. This procedure is called an **episiotomy (eh PEEZ ee OT oh mee)**. There is some controversy about whether it is needed as frequently as it is performed.

BREASTS

The breasts (see Figure 24) are also considered part of the female reproductive system because their primary function is to produce milk to nourish the young. They are located in the front of the chest over the pectoral muscles, and do not develop until puberty. The breasts are made up of adipose, or fatty, tissue and the **mammary (MAM er ee) glands,** which lactate **(LACK tate)** (secrete milk). The adipose tissue determines the size of the breasts, and serves as a protective padding for the system of glands and ducts beneath it.

Mammary Glands
The mammary glands are in the form of alveoli **(al VEE oh ly),** or grape-like clusters that would remind you of the structures that exchange oxygen and carbon dioxide in the lungs. Ducts transport the milk from the alveoli to the main duct, called the **lactiferous (lack TIF er uss) duct,** which leads directly to the nipple. The alveoli are grouped in 15 to 20 sections of the breast

---

ORGASM AND PREGNANCY

Stimulation of the clitoris produces orgasm. You may have heard that the contractions of the pelvic muscles during orgasm help push the sperm upward toward the egg and the uterus. However, there is no medical proof that orgasm has any effect on reproduction.

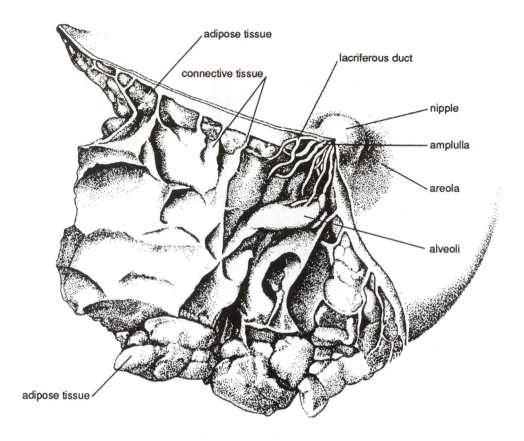

Labels on figure: adipose tissue, connective tissue, lacriferous duct, nipple, amplulla, areola, alveoli, adipose tissue

Figure 24: Female breast, anterior view.

called lobes. The lobes are separated from each other by walls made of connective tissue and lined with adipose tissue. Each lobe has one lactiferous duct, and all the alveoli in that section empty into the single duct. Each duct ends in a small opening on the surface of the nipple. Just before it reaches the nipple, each duct widens slightly to form a reservoir for extra milk.

Areola and Nipple

On the surface of the breast, the nipple is surrounded by the **areola (ah REE oh lah),** a circular area of pigment darker than the surrounding skin. The nipple is the same color as the areola. In light-skinned women, the areola and nipple darken from pink to brown in the first pregnancy, and remain brownish from then on. No comparable change occurs in dark-skinned women.

Lymph Vessels

Lymph vessels are found throughout the breasts. These vessels do two things: They drain extra fluid from spaces between the cells. They also pick up protein and other molecules that need to be returned to the blood, either because they have been lost from the blood vessels during the exchange of nutrients and wastes, or because they are foreign bodies that need to be eliminated from the circulation by the white blood cells.

The lymph vessels in the breasts are interconnected and drain into the pectoral muscles. Through this system, breast cancers travel throughout the breast and into the chest wall. This interconnectivity is why breast cancer is so dangerous, and why the chest muscles sometimes are removed with a cancerous breast to be sure that all potentially diseased tissue is eliminated.

MENSTRUAL CYCLE

The menstrual cycle is a complex series of events involving the ovaries, uterus, vagina, pituitary gland, and breasts. The cycle prepares the body for ovum fertilization and implantation. If this occurs, the cycle stops until after childbirth. It then resumes. If fertilization does not interrupt the cycle, the cycle is completed at the beginning of the menstrual period.

The menstrual cycle occurs throughout much of a woman's life. It begins with **menarche (meh NAR kee),** or the first menstrual period in puberty, usually at about age 13, and continues to menopause, or the last period, at about age 45 to 50. An average woman can expect to menstruate approximately 480 times, depending on the number of pregnancies. The cycle lasts an average of 28 to 30 days.

The length and regularity of the menstrual cycle differ from woman to woman and within each woman's lifetime. Changes in cycle length and skipping an occasional cycle altogether are normal and unpredictable. The cycle may be affected by outside events, such as emotional stress, a job change, moving from one home to another, a vacation, a new school term, or any of a number of other events that could influence hormonal activity. Women who exercise strenuously often experience **amenorrhea (ah MEN of REE ah),** or absence of menses. Apparently the menstrual cycle ceases if body fat is not sufficient to provide energy for the woman and the developing fetus. Amenorrhea can also accompany other stressful situations. Some variations in the menstrual cycle are caused by disease. These will be discussed in Chapter 6.

This complicated series of delicately interrelated events is more easily understood if it can be studied against a background of time. The first day of the menses, which begins the shedding of the uterine lining, generally is referred to as Day 1 of the menstrual cycle. Because the onset of the menses is an event that can be pinpointed with accuracy, it marks the beginning of each menstrual cycle.

Hormonal Influences

The rise and fall of four different hormones produce different phases during the 28- to 30-day menstrual cycle (see Figure 25). Before describing the different phases of the normal menstrual cycle, it is helpful to discuss which hormones rise and fall to produce these changes (see Table 5).

Follicle stimulating hormone (FSH) and **luteinizing hormone** (LH) are released by the anterior pituitary gland which is vital to reproduction. The pituitary gland lies on the underside of the brain and produces many different hormones. (For a more thorough discussion of the pituitary gland, its function and hormones, see the book on endocrinology in this series.) In very young women, FSH and LH stimulate the development of the first ovarian follicles. It may be some time after the initial onset of puberty before a full menstrual cycle is completed. A regular pattern of menstruation might not be present for several months.

Estrogen is secreted from the ovarian follicle. Estrogen is also responsible for the development of the secondary sex characteristics and maturation of the external reproductive organs. Progesterone is secreted from the corpus luteum.

Three Phases of the Menstrual Cycle

Using hormonal activity as a guide, the menstrual cycle can be studied in three phases. The **menstrual phase** (also called menses or

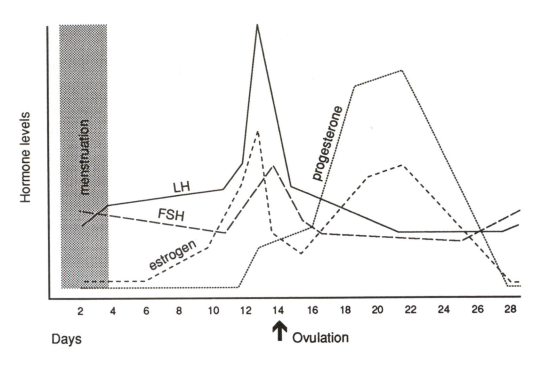

Figure 25: The rise and fall of hormone levels during the menstrual cycle.

Table 5: Sex Hormones and Their Origin and Roles in the Menstrual Cycle

Hormone	Function	Produced by
Follicle-Stimulating Hormone (FSH)	Stimulates growth of ovarian follicle, which then produces estrogen, stimulates ovulation	Anterior pituitary gland
Estrogen	Initiates thickening of endometrium, stimulates production of LH, stimulates development of breasts and other secondary sex characteristics at puberty	Ovarian follicle Corpus luteum
Luteinizing Hormone (LH)	Stimulates completion of follicle growth, ovulation and growth of corpus luteum	Anterior pituitary gland
Progesterone	Promotes preparation of endometrium to receive embryo	Corpus luteum

period) occurs when the endometrium is shed. The **follicular phase** occurs when hormones stimulate the ovarian follicles, and the follicles actively secrete estrogen. The **luteal phase** occurs when the ruptured follicle becomes the corpus luteum and begins to secrete progesterone. These phases often overlap and vary in different women and at different stages of life. Figure 26 shows the relationship between egg growth and the growth of the uterine lining. These are all caused by hormone activity.

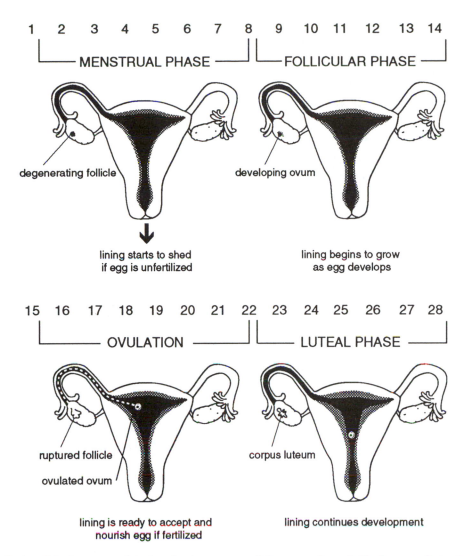

1 2 3 4 5 6 7 8 9 10 11 12 13 14

MENSTRUAL PHASE — FOLLICULAR PHASE

degenerating follicle

developing ovum

lining starts to shed
if egg is unfertilized

lining begins to grow
as egg develops

15 16 17 18 19 20 21 22 23 24 25 26 27 28

OVULATION — LUTEAL PHASE

ruptured follicle
ovulated ovum

corpus luteum

lining is ready to accept and
nourish egg if fertilized

lining continues development

Figure 26: Relationship between the developing egg and the growth and discharge of uterine lining.

Menstrual Phase. During this phase, which lasts for 2 to 8 days, the uterus sheds part of the endometrium. The arterioles (tiny spiral-shaped arteries in the deep layer of the endometrium) constrict, and the cells in the outer lining of the uterus die from lack of oxygen and other nutrients. The superficial and middle layers of the endometrium are shed. The pituitary gland increases FHS secretion, causing several ovarian follicles in one ovary to begin to develop.

Follicular Phase. Ovarian follicles grow and begin to secrete estrogen. The pituitary increases LH secretion slowly. Estrogen and FSH encourage the oogonium within the follicle to mature and ripen.

Estrogen also causes the growth of blood vessels and the thickening of the superficial layer of the endometrium. Cells multiply and elongate; the arterioles infiltrate the newly formed and expanded tissue. The tissue also retains extra fluid, which further increases its thickness.

As the ovum matures, an increased level of LH from the pituitary ruptures the **graafian follicle (GRAY fee an FOL lick ul)** or **vesicular ovarian follicle** (ripe ovarian follicle). The ovum passes out of the ovary and into the abdominal cavity. This is called **ovulation**. The ovum is pulled by the fimbriae into the uterine tube and slowly migrates toward the uterus. It requires about 5 days for the ovum to travel from the ruptured follicle to the uterus.

Luteal Phase. Under the influence of LH from the pituitary gland, the ruptured follicle becomes a hormone-secreting gland called the corpus luteum. The corpus luteum begins to secrete estrogen and progesterone. The follicles that did not mature quickly enough disintegrate.

Progesterone from the corpus luteum causes blood vessels in the functional layer of the endometrium to grow and start to collect nutrients for use in the event an egg is fertilized. If this happens, the corpus luteum remains in the ovary and secretes hormones for 4 to 5 months.

As progesterone levels increase, LH levels decrease. If the ovum is not fertilized, the corpus luteum gradually stops secreting hormones and disintegrates. Without progesterone, the endometrium stops growing and begins to slough off, and the menstrual cycle begins again with menses.

MENOPAUSE

After some 35 years of menstrual cycles, the pituitary gland releases decreasing amounts of FSH and LH, and the ovaries produce less estrogen and progesterone. Menstrual cycles become increasing irregular and eventually stop altogether.

The cessation of the menstrual cycle is called the menopause. Menopause is a natural event in the life of every woman. Most women begin menopause in their late forties, and menstrual periods have usually ended by the midfifties. Individuals vary, however. A woman may enter menopause earlier or much later. Each woman responds to the changing biochemical rhythms of menopause in a different way. About 25 percent of women have no symptoms except for amenorrhea. Some women, on the other hand are deeply affected physically and emotionally.

Physical symptoms may include sweating, hot flashes, urinary problems, joint pain, headache, vaginal dryness that may make sexual intercourse uncomfortable, palpitations (irregular heartbeat), irritability, depression, anxiety, problems with concentration, sleeplessness, or loss of self-confidence. In addition, some women may worry about growing old, and no longer being able to conceive and bear children.

Symptoms of menopause can last for as long as 5 years, or only a few weeks or months. However, they usually last for 12 to 18 months.

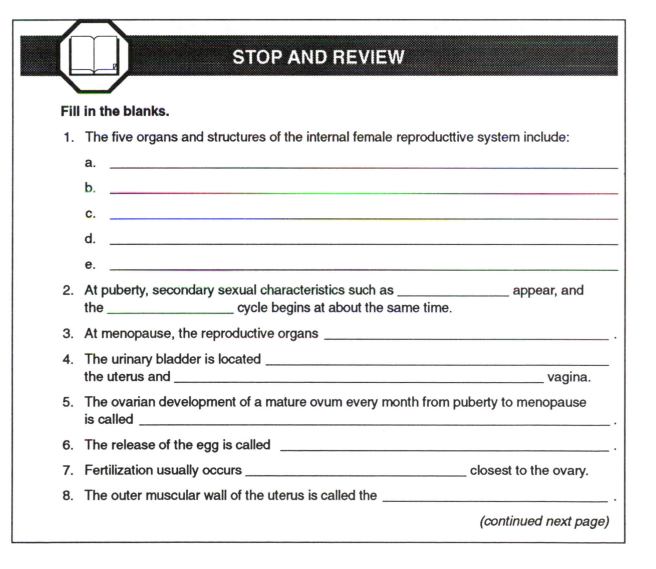

STOP AND REVIEW

Fill in the blanks.

1. The five organs and structures of the internal female reproducttive system include:

   a. _____

   b. _____

   c. _____

   d. _____

   e. _____

2. At puberty, secondary sexual characteristics such as _____ appear, and the _____ cycle begins at about the same time.

3. At menopause, the reproductive organs _____ .

4. The urinary bladder is located _____ the uterus and _____ vagina.

5. The ovarian development of a mature ovum every month from puberty to menopause is called _____ .

6. The release of the egg is called _____ .

7. Fertilization usually occurs _____ closest to the ovary.

8. The outer muscular wall of the uterus is called the _____ .

   (continued next page)

STOP AND REVIEW

9. The vagina is a tube located behind the _____ and in front of the _____ .

10. The external female genitals, collectively, are called the _____ .

11. An episiotomy is a surgical procedure to cut the _____ during delivery.

12. The breasts are made up of _____ glands together with adipose tissue, which functions as _____ .

13. The reservoirs for extra milk, just before the nipple, are called _____ .

14. The menstrual cycle includes three phases:

    a. _____

    b. _____

    c. _____

15. The shedding of the _____ lining is also known as menses.

16. The follicle out of which the mature ovum passes or ovulates is called the _____ follicle.

17. The _____ of the fallopian tube "catch" the ovulated ovum.

18. The _____ gland secretes FSH and LH.

19. Human chorionic gonadotropin signals the _____ to release progesterone, which keeps the uterus lining thick and ready to receive the embryo.

Short answers

20. Describe three differences between the male and female pelvis:

    a. _____

    b. _____

    c. _____

21. List two functions of the uterus.

    a. _____

    b. _____

22. Identify three major functions of the vagina.

    a. _____

    b. _____

    c. _____

23. Describe the function of the lymph vessels in the breast.

    _____

    _____

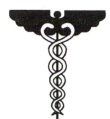
Knowledge Objectives

After completing this chapter, you should be able to:

- describe some disorders of the menstrual cycle
- list three sexually transmitted diseases and their symptoms in women
- describe some common disorders of the menstrual cycle
- describe three common uterine displacements
- describe two benign and two malignant growths of the female reproductive system and discuss how each one is treated
- list and describe four nonsurgical diagnostic examinations of the female reproductive system and their frequency

Disorders of the Female Reproductive System

The female reproductive system is susceptible to the same sorts of disorders of its structures, organs, or cycles as the male. These include infections, abnormal growths, blockages, and chemical and hormonal imbalances. The female reproductive organs are seldom injured, however, because they are protected within the pelvic girdle.

DISORDERS OF THE MENSTRUAL CYCLE

The menstrual cycle may be disrupted by a number of causes, which may or may not involve disease. Such disruptions can cause temporary or permanent infertility. Disorders related to pregnancy and childbirth will be covered in Chapter 7.

Amenorrhea

This term means absence of menstrual periods. It is a normal condition before menarche and after menopause. It also is normal in pregnancy, when the lining of the uterus is retained instead of being shed because it is needed to nurture the growing fetus. In the 8 months after conception, ovulation does not occur and the cycle is temporarily halted.

In a woman who is not pregnant, amenorrhea does not necessarily mean the woman is not ovulating. This is important to remember if a patient wishes to avoid pregnancy. Even if ovulation does stop, it can begin again at any time.

Amenorrhea can be caused by a strenuous athletic training program, extreme weight loss, an emotional upset or stress, or even fear of pregnancy. Amenorrhea in a woman of childbearing age usually does not require treatment. If the patient is not pregnant and does not have other symptoms that suggest a disorder, the periods will probably resume within a few months.

Dysmenorrhea

Dysmenorrhea (DIS men oh REE ah) means painful periods, or menstrual cramps. Many women have mild dysmenorrhea in the first few years of menstruation, before the cycle is well established. Others have cramps until their first child is born or throughout the childbearing years. Menstrual pain can occur due to using an intrauterine device (IUD) for contraception. Mild dysmenorrhea can be relieved with use of acetaminophen or other nonprescription pain medications. Severe pain should be evaluated by a doctor to identify an underlying problem, such as endometriosis or pelvic infection.

Oligomenorrhea

This term means infrequent periods. **Oligomenorrhea (OL ih goh MEN oh REE ah)** often is a part of menopause, but it can also occur because of a different hormonal cycle. Usually no treatment is necessary.

PREMENSTRUAL SYNDROME (PMS)

Premenstrual syndrome refers to symptoms such as unusual irritability, aggressiveness, or depression occurring with cramping, fluid retention, breast tenderness, and sometimes headaches which occur before the onset of menses. The exact cause of PMS is unknown. It may be related to decreasing estrogen and progesterone levels. However, other factors, such as vitamin deficiencies and psychological disturbances have not been ruled out.

Diagnosis is usually made after three consecutive menstrual cycles in which the same symptoms occur. The week just before the menstrual period when estrogen and progesterone secretion reaches a peak and then ceases is the time when symptoms occur. At the same time, the patient may feel physically uncomfortable, with cramping, fluid retention, breast tenderness, and sometimes headaches.

Sometimes dietary changes, exercise, or mild medication therapy will provide relief. In extreme cases, the doctor may prescribe diuretics or oral contraceptives, which consist of artificial estrogen and progesterone, to balance the cycle. This can help to reduce mood changes and make them more manageable.

INFECTIONS

All parts of the female reproductive system are subject to infection, including the breasts, vagina, vulva, and interior pelvic area. These infections can be caused by bacteria, viruses, fungi, or parasites. Some are transmitted by sexual contact. Others can be contracted from organisms that are normally found in the body in small numbers (normal flora), but that may increase in number because of changes in the body, and then cause disease. Still others come from the environment.

Sexually Transmitted Diseases (STD's)

These diseases are passed from person to person by sexual contact. Their symptoms and treatment were discussed in Chapter 4. Most of the symptoms of the STDs described below relate to women specifically.

Acquired Immune Deficiency Syndrome (AIDS).

Acquired immune deficiency syndrome (AIDS) is becoming an increasing problem for women and their infants. AIDS is commonly caused by the human immunodeficiency virus (HIV). Sexual transmission was discussed in Chapter 4 and is described in detail in the book on immunology in this series. Statistics indicate that 75 percent of women who are infected with HIV are of childbearing age. Because AIDS can be transmitted across the placental barrier, during birth, or in breast milk, increasing numbers of infants are born infected with HIV. AIDS in women is now spreading quickly in heterosexual women, so it is certain that AIDS will continue to be an area of needed research.

Chlamydial Infections.
Several strains of chlamydia cause genital and urinary infections in women and infants born to infected mothers. The disease is the greatest cause of pel-

vic inflammatory disease (PID), resulting in severe urethritis and infertility. Women often carry the infection without symptoms, and continue to infect partners and offspring.

Gonorrhea. In a woman, the cervix is usually the original site of gonorrhea infection, so there may be no outward signs of the disease. Symptoms may not occur or may include a cloudy vaginal discharge, abdominal discomfort, bleeding, or painful urination. The vestibular glands at the opening of the vagina and the paraurethral glands at the urethral opening are often affected if the infection spreads. They become swollen, tender, and later abscessed. If gonorrhea is not treated, it can spread to the uterus and fallopian tubes and can cause infertility or ectopic pregnancy (pregnancy that occurs in a location other than the uterus).

Diagnosis and treatment were discussed in the section on STDs in Chapter 4. The infant of an infected mother may have acute inflammation of the conjunctiva. The gonococci enter the infant's eyes during delivery, and if the cornea becomes infected, blindness results. To prevent this infection, a drop of silver nitrate is routinely placed in the eyes of newborns.

Syphilis. The symptoms, diagnosis, and treatment of syphilis are the same in men and women. In addition, the infant of an infected mother may be born with syphilis. Congenital defects may include deformities, mental retardation, and deafness or blindness. A fetus may die or spontaneously abort in the presence of syphilis infection.

Genital Herpes. Aside from being inconvenient and painful, genital herpes in women can be dangerous to the fetus if the infection is active during childbirth. Spontaneous abortion or premature delivery can occur as it passes through the birth canal. The infection can spread to the fetus, and can cause serious problems, including an eye infection that can lead to blindness. A cesarean delivery may be done to reduce the risk of infection in the infant.

Hepatitis B. Hepatitis B was discussed in Chapter 4. The symptoms, diagnosis, and treatment are the same for women. It is important to repeat that the virus can be transmitted from mother to infant during birth. Vaccination against hepatitis B may become part of routine newborn immunization.

Genital Warts (Condylomata Acuminata).
Caused by the human papilloma virus, genital warts are fibrous tissue growths on the vulva, vagina, and cervix. They multiply rapidly over the perianal region. The virus reached epidemic proportions during the 1980s. Although clearly an STD, it is currently not reported to public health authorities. Many times it is accompanied by other STDs. The warts cause itching, irritation, and occasional bleeding, and they are likely to become infected. Studies have also suggested a connection between genital warts and increased incidence of cervical cancer.

Some warts may spontaneously disappear without medical treatment, but it may be necessary to them. If a wart is small, topical drug therapy can be effective. If the wart is large, surgery, cryosurgery, electrocoagulation, or laser vaporization may be necessary. Sexual partners must also be treated. Even with treatment, condylomas recur in at least 20 percent of patients.

Other Infections
Vaginitis. Infections of the vagina are very common and have several possible causes.

Trichomoniasis (TRICK oh moh NY ah sis) and **candidiasis** (KAN dih DY ah sis) are seen most often. The trichomonad is a parasite, and the candida is a yeast. The symptoms of both infections include burning, itching, irritation, an abnormal discharge from the vagina, and sometimes pain or discomfort during sexual intercourse or during urination. The discharge of trichomoniasis is yellowish-green and has an unpleasant odor. Candidiasis causes a thick, white discharge.

Trichomoniasis can be transmitted by sexual contact, but it does not cause any symptoms in the man. A patient's sexual partner should be treated for the problem at the same time that she is, or she will probably be reinfected. The yeast that causes candidiasis is a normal inhabitant of the reproductive organs. It causes problems when the acid balance of the vagina is upset and the organisms reproduce too rapidly. The balance is upset when acid-producing bacteria in the vagina are killed by broad-spectrum antibiotics or too-frequent use of commercial douches or vaginal sprays. Use of birth control pills can also upset the acid balance of the vagina. Pregnancy and diabetes mellitus make women more susceptible to candida infections.

These infections can usually be diagnosed by observing the discharge under a microscope. The two causative organisms have distinctive appearances. Trichomonads have tails called flagellae, and they move across the visual field. Yeasts stay in one place and may have buds, or tiny rounded projections, on the cells. Sometimes a culture must be grown to identify the causative organism.

Trichomoniasis is treated with an oral medication prescribed for both sexual partners. Candidiasis is treated with an antifungal drug prepared in suppository or cream form, which is inserted directly into the vagina.

Salpingitis. Salpingitis (SAL pin JY tis) is inflammation of the uterine tubes caused by untreated gonorrhea or a streptococcal or staphylococcal infection. The uterine tubes become red and swollen, and infection can spread to the pelvic cavity. The tubes can close and fill with pus. Both tubes are usually affected and sterility can result. Salpingitis can cause menstrual abnormalities and ectopic pregnancy. Infection subsides with antibiotic treatment.

Toxic Shock Syndrome (TSS). **Toxic shock syndrome** is an acute bacterial infection that usually occurs in menstruating women who are using tampons (particularly superabsorbent tampons). Women at risk for TSS are those who insert tampons with their fingers, those with chronic vaginal infections, and those with genital herpes. TSS has also been diagnosed in nonmenstruating women and even in men. In these cases it has been associated with cellulitis (an inflammation of the connective tissue), surgical wound infections, and subcutaneous abscesses.

The symptoms are flu-like during the first 24 hours. Then, between the second and third days of the menstrual cycle, the patient has a spiking fever (up to 39° C), experiences vomiting, diarrhea, hypotension, and signs of septic shock (shock produced by an overwhelming infection). Sore throat, headache, and rash may be followed by decreased urinary output and finally disorientation.

Blood, urine, and vaginal cultures are evaluated to confirm the diagnosis and pinpoint the causative organism. Treatment corresponds to the causative bacteria and the severity of the symptoms. Antibiotics are prescribed and fluid and electrolyte replacement may be indicated if severe dehydration results from vomiting and diarrhea. When vaginal cultures are negative and the patient no longer has any of the signs and symptoms of TSS, she is taught the following preventive measures:

- Avoid using tampons until cleared by the physician
- Wash hands before using a tampon
- Avoid using high-absorbency tampons
- Change tampons frequently during the day and wear a sanitary napkin at night
- Immediately report any recurrence of symptoms

Pelvic Inflammatory Disease (PID). A pelvic infection is one that affects the entire pelvic area, including the vagina, uterus, fallopian tubes, ovaries, and the tissues around them. It is called **pelvic inflammatory disease** (PID). Some possible causes are untreated STDs or other infections. Miscarriage or an abortion in which sterile procedures were not followed can also cause PID. Also, use of an IUD increases the possibility of a generalized pelvic infection. The symptoms may include mild to severe pain in the lower abdomen, painful intercourse, fever, heavy or irregular menstrual flow, and sometimes an abnormal and offensive vaginal discharge.

It is often difficult to identify the causative organism of PID. An antibiotic is usually prescribed, along with bed rest, fluids, and pain relievers. If the problem does not clear, further tests will be necessary and hospitalization may be required until the cause of the infection can be identified and treated.

Vulvitis. **Vulvitis (vul VY tis)** means inflammation of the vulva. The vaginal and venereal infections described earlier may cause swelling, itching, and discomfort in the vulva. Rashes, sores, ulcers, warts and other skin eruptions can also occur on the vulva as a result of these diseases. The treatment depends on the cause. Usually an antibiotic drug or a cream or lotion applied to the area, or both, will cure the infection.

Breast Abscess (Mastitis). The breasts are also susceptible to infection, especially in women who are breast-feeding. Infection usually enters through the nipple and causes an abscess, or pocket of pus, in one or more milk ducts. The abscess is usually very painful. The lymph glands under the arm may also be swollen and painful, and the patient may have a fever.

Mastitis (mas TY tis) is usually treated with antibiotics. If the infection does not resolve, the abscess may have to be drained by making a small cut in the nipple. The patient should continue to breastfeed.

ENDOMETRIOSIS

This disorder occurs when endometrial tissue grows in locations other than the inner lining of the uterus. The most common site for **endometriosis (EN doh MEE tree OH sis),** is the ovaries, but other parts of the pelvic area—including the large intestine—can be involved. This extraneous tissue grows and sheds with the menstrual cycle, causing an accumulation of dead cells and blood wherever it is located. This may cause pain (usually at menstruation), painful intercourse, and abnormal vaginal bleeding. It may also cause infertility. In some cases, however, it causes no symptoms. It is not known exactly how or why the endometrial tissue grows in these locations. Endometriosis is most common in women from age 30 to 40. It often improves during pregnancy and may disappear after delivery.

Treatment of endometriosis depends on

the severity of the symptoms and the patient's desire to have children. In severe cases, if the patient is near menopause and does not intend to have children, **hysterectomy (HIS teh RECK toh mee**; surgical removal of the uterus), and possibly removal of the ovaries and fallopian tubes as well, may be recommended. In other cases, surgery done by video laseroscopy (a video camera with laser) can often remove most tissue. For mild cases, pain relievers may be sufficient treatment. Steroid hormones, including estrogen, progesterone, or androgens (male hormones), may be prescribed when symptoms are more severe and the patient wishes to have children.

INFERTILITY

Some women would like to have children but cannot become pregnant. In such cases, the woman and her husband or sexual partner should be tested and treated. Usually the man's sperm count is measured first (see Chapter 4). If he is fertile, the woman is examined to detect any hormone imbalance, dysfunction of the ovaries, blockage or other problems in the uterine tubes, or uterine incompatibility (the inability of the uterus to hold and nourish the fertilized egg).

Diagnosis of infertility includes a test of the cervical mucus and sperm count after intercourse, called the post-coital test, and an x-ray study called **hysterosalpingography (his ter oh sal ping GOG roh fee),** in which a dye is introduced into the reproductive system to detect blockage of the tubes and uterine abnormalities. If the woman's periods are irregular, ovulation can be monitored by keeping records of daily body temperature and by a biopsy of the endometrium.

If the cause of infertility can be found,

there are a number of treatments that can be tried to allow the patient to become pregnant. If the problem is caused by hormone imbalances, the doctor may prescribe fertility drugs or hormone replacement drugs. Blockages can sometimes be removed surgically. If necessary, the couple may be referred to an infertility clinic for additional testing or special procedures, such as in vitro fertilization or gamete intrafallopian transfer.

UTERINE DISPLACEMENTS

Since the uterus's normal position is at right angles to the vagina, uterine displacement means that it is not in this normal anatomical position (see Figure 27). Most uterine displacements are simple and have no clinical significance. **Retroversion (RET roh VUR zhun),** a turning backward of the uterus, is the most common displacement and may be brought about by childbirth.

Uterine displacements that are caused by a weakening of the pelvic muscles may also have varying degrees of flexion. Diagnosis is made by pelvic examination and x-ray films.

Uterine Prolapse

When the pelvic muscles that support the uterus atrophy or weaken, they no longer can maintain the uterus in its normal position. The uterus may then collapse into the vagina (see Figure 27). This is called a **uterine prolapse (PROH laps)**. It may cause urinary incontinence or retention, constipation, backache, or vaginal discharge. These symptoms may be made worse by coughing or prolonged standing.

Treatment is done by using a **pessary (PES ah ree),** a device that is inserted into the vagina to support the uterus and correct the displacement. This is the usual treatment for a woman who cannot withstand surgery.

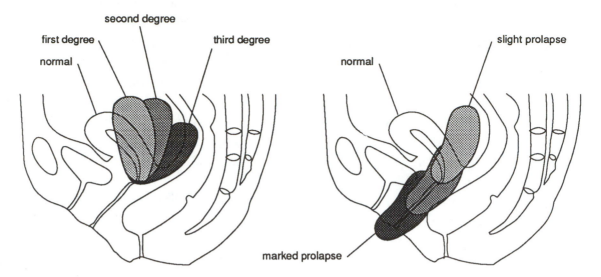

THE THREE DEGREES
OF RETROVERSION

second degree

first degree

third degree

normal

UTERINE
PROLAPSE

slight prolapse

normal

marked prolapse

Figure 27: Uterine retroversion and prolapse.

However, hysterectomy is the preferred treatment in an older woman.

Cystocele

A **cystocele (SIS toh seel)** is a protrusion of the bladder into the vaginal vault. It is caused by weak pelvic muscles and usually accompanied by symptoms such as urinary frequency and urgency and stress incontinence. Diagnosis is made by visual inspection during a pelvic examination.

Correction is done surgically by tightening the pelvic muscles that support the bladder. The surgery is called anterior colporrhaphy **(kol POR ah fee)** and is done vaginally.

Rectocele

A **rectocele (RECK toh seel)** is a protrusion of the rectum into the vaginal vault. This condition is accompanied by rectal pressure, constipation, feelings of heaviness, and hemorrhoids. Diagnosis is made on pelvic examination or x-ray films of the lower bowel. Surgery to strengthen the weakened muscles is called a posterior colporrhaphy and is often done with an anterior colporrhaphy.

ABNORMAL GROWTHS

Abnormal growths can occur in any part of the female reproductive system and can be benign or malignant. Benign growths do not spread to other parts of the body and generally do not damage adjoining tissue. They usually do not cause symptoms, unless their position or size interferes with normal body functions. Malignant growths are also called cancerous growths. They tend to metastasize, or spread to other parts of the body. They also can damage surrounding tissue. If untreated, malignant growths are life-threatening, while most benign growths are not.

Benign Growths

Ovarian Cyst. A cyst, or fluid-filled sac of tissue, can form on an ovary as well as in breast tissue. Some ovarian cysts form in an ovarian follicle and disappear within 1 month just as a normal follicle in a normal menstrual cycle would do. These cysts seldom cause symptoms or require treatment. Other types of ovarian cysts can grow quite large, and in some cases may interfere with ovarian function, or may cause pain during intercourse. Occasionally, a cyst will rupture or become twisted, which will cause abdominal pain and sometimes bleeding. A ruptured cyst can cause **peritonitis (PER ih toh NY tis),** or infection of the abdominal cavity.

The physician diagnoses a cyst by sonography or **laparoscopy (LAP ah ROS koh pee)** (examining the ovary with an instrument called a laparoscope. Sometimes a biopsy is also necessary to verify that the growth is not malignant. A cyst that is large enough to be felt or that interferes with ovarian function will usually be drained or surgically removed. Sometimes it is necessary to remove the entire ovary and the fallopian tube on that side.

Fibroids.   Another term for benign tumors of the uterus—called **fibroids (FY broydz)**—is **myoma (my OH mah).** They generally do not cause symptoms, and may be discovered by accident when the physician treats the patient for a different problem. Fibroids can grow quite large, however. Some are large enough to mimic a pregnancy, and fill the uterus completely. Others grow in the lower part of the uterus and press on the bladder or urethra, causing frequent or painful urination.

Fibroids are very common, especially in women over age 40. The physician can usually diagnose this type of growth by palpation of the uterus. If it is necessary to remove one or more fibroids, a surgical procedure called a **myomectomy (MY oh MECK toh mee)** is used. Sometimes, if the tumor is very large, if it is inaccessible, if the patient has other problems such as ovarian tumors, or if the patient is past menopause, the physician may recommend hysterectomy.

Cervical Erosion and Cervical Dysplasia.   These two conditions are related because **cervical erosion** can lead to **cervical dysplasia (dis PLAY see ah).** In cervical erosion, the type of tissue that lines the uterus (columnar epithelium) grows over the cervix, which normally is covered with squamous epithelium. This change in tissue type may cause an abnormal discharge, and the area may be abnormally susceptible to infection. Otherwise, the condition usually does not cause problems. In cervical dysplasia, abnormal cells develop on the cervix, in the same location where cervical erosion has occurred. These cells do not cause any symptoms, but may gradually (over 10 to 15 years) develop into cervical cancer.

Because dysplasia is an early sign of cancer, physicians test for it regularly. The **Papanicolaou (PAP ah NICK oh LAY oh),** or Pap, smear is used as a screening test for this condition. If the Pap smear shows abnormal cells on the cervix, the physician uses a **colposcope (KOL poh skohp)** to examine the cervix, and may take a sample of tissue for a biopsy, to be sure no cancer is present. The abnormal cells may be removed after the cells from the biopsy have been analyzed by a pathologist. Heat (cauterization) **(KAW ter ih ZAY shun),** freezing (cryotherapy; **KRY oh THER ah pee),** or laser can be used to remove them. If the dysplasia covers a large area, the physician may recommend a cone biopsy to remove more tissue. This procedure may require hospitalization. Colposcopy can be done in a medical office.

A patient who has had cervical dysplasia should have frequent (two to four per year) Pap smears done for several years to be sure the condition does not recur and eventually become malignant.

Cervical Polyps.   Polyps are small, benign growths. **Cervical polyps (POL ips)** are made up of mucus-producing tissue, and can cause an abnormal bloody and watery discharge. The symptoms resemble those of cervical cancer. Polyps are not dangerous, but they should be examined to be sure cancer is not involved. A Pap smear is used to detect any abnormal cells. Treatment involves removing the growths (usually an easy procedure that can be done in the physician's office).

Benign Breast Disease. Lumps in the breasts can be perfectly normal, though newly noted lumps can be benign or malignant. The cause of benign breast disease is unknown although some evidence suggests it is related to the hormonal pattern. Three of the most common of these diseases are: **fibrocystic (FY broh SIS tick) disease**, **fiboadenoma (FY broh AD eh NOH mah)**, and **mammary duct ectasia (eck TAY zee ah)**.

Fibrocystic disease is the most common benign breast disease. It is characterized by lumpy breasts, tenderness, and sometimes nipple discharge. It produces a lump, called a cyst, which is a soft, movable, fluid-filled sac of tissue. These cysts may be single or multiple.

Any new breast lump should be evaluated for possible malignancy. Diagnosis is based on physical examination and the patient's history. Mammography or ultrasonography can be used to rule out a solid tumor. Usually the physician will aspirate the fluid in the lump to determine whether malignant cells are present. If the lump aspirate contains no malignant cells, follow-up usually involves regular repeat mammograms and clinical examinations. The physician may also prescribe hormones if the lump is tender or painful. If its recurs and repeat aspirations are not effective, a surgical excision of the lump may be performed, or in rare instances partial **mastectomy (mas TECK toh mee)**.

A **fibroadenoma** is the second most common benign breast tumor. It is the most common tumor in women under age 25 and is related to the hormonal changes of menarche, specifically, a thickening of the milk glands in the breast. These tumors are firm, round, and movable with clear edges. They are influenced by the menstrual cycle, increasing in size before menstruation and pregnancy.

Diagnosis is made by physical examination, history, and mammography. Medication and dietary changes do not seem to affect the condition in any way. Excision of a lump may be done if the symptoms are severe or the doctor suspects that the fibroadenoma may become malignant.

Mammary duct ectasia begins with duct inflammation, which resolves but is followed by duct hardening and enlargement. In a premenopausal woman, this is accompanied by breast pain, a palpable mass, and a thick, sticky nipple discharge. There may also be itching and pain under the areola before menses. A postmenopausal woman has nipple retraction as a result of duct hardening. Mammary duct ectasia usually requires no treatment. If the ducts become infected or if an abscess develops, an antibiotic will be ordered and the abscess will be drained.

Malignant Growths

Cancerous growths can occur in the breasts, ovaries, uterus, or vulva. In women, breast cancer is the most common form of malignancy. Cervical cancer is the third most common cancer of the female reproductive system. As with other types of cancer, early detection and prompt treatment greatly increase the patient's chances of cure. Treatment is as for other types of cancer: surgical removal of the tumor, radiation therapy, and chemotherapy are used alone, or more commonly in combination, to try to eliminate the malignant growth before it can metastasize.

Cervical Cancer. Cancer of the cervix is one of the cancers most easily diagnosed in its early stages. Since the development of the Pap smear, its incidence has significantly decreased.

If, however, a Pap smear and a follow-up biopsy show cancerous cells on the cervix, the diagnosis of cervical cancer is made. The physician may also do a dilatation and curettage (D&C) to learn whether the cancer has spread to the uterus. Treatment of cervical cancer depends on the patient's age and her desire to have children. In a young woman who wants to to have children, **conization (KON ih ZAY shun)** of the cervix may be performed. In this procedure a cone-shaped sample of tissue is removed from the cervix. In other cases, a hysterectomy may be necessary. In cases of invasive cervical cancer, the tubes and ovaries will also be removed, and this will be followed by radiation therapy. If the cancer has not spread, the likelihood of complete recovery is very high.

Cancer of the cervix seems to follow chronic irritation, infection, and poor hygiene. Promiscuity at an early age involving many partners seems somehow related to this cancer.

Ovarian Cancer. Malignant growths on the ovaries are uncommon, but difficult to detect in early stages. The ovaries are far from the surface of the abdomen, so small swellings often are not detected. Ovarian cancer does not generally cause symptoms until the later stages of the disease. These symptoms include fluid accumulation in the abdominal cavity, which is called **ascites (ah SY teez),** and also abdominal pain and weight loss. Treatment usually involves removal of the uterus, both fallopian tubes,

both ovaries, and the omentum (protective fatty tissue in the abdomen). Adjacent lymph glands may also have to be removed, depending on whether the cancer has spread. Surgery is usually followed by radiation, chemotherapy, or both.

Cancer of the Uterus. A malignant growth in the uterus often starts in the endometrium. From there, it spreads first to the uterine wall and then to the other reproductive organs. The growth causes abnormal vaginal bleeding and pain similar to menstrual cramps. Diagnosis and treatment are the same as for cervical cancer. Radiation treatment may be given by implanting a radium capsule in the vagina. The capsule releases small doses of radiation over time.

Cancer of the Vulva. This form of cancer produces a lump on the vulva that becomes an ulcer. The ulcer may ooze or bleed, and grows very slowly. Diagnosis is made by a biopsy of the ulcer. Treatment is by removal of the growth and the adjacent tissue, which is called a **vulvectomy (vul VECK toh mee).** Sometimes the lymph glands in the groin must be removed as well. Radiation therapy may be needed as a follow-up to surgery.

Breast Cancer. Breast cancer appears as lumps in the breast. Many cancers and benign breast growths are discovered by patients who examine their breasts regularly to detect new breasts lumps or changes. Other symptoms are retracted nipples and skin dimples on the breast.

Breast cancer is a particularly dangerous form of malignancy because of the network of lymph vessels in the breasts. This network provides a pathway that malignant cells can follow to other parts of the body, especially the lymph nodes.

Single women, women who have borne

no children, and women with a family history of breast cancer seem more likely than others to develop cancer of the breast. This cancer usually develops at about the time of menopause and appears to be related to estrogen activity.

Mammography can detect small cancers early. It should be recommended according to age. A biopsy of the tissue confirms the diagnosis or proves the tumor to be benign.

Treatment of breast cancer almost always requires surgical removal of the tumor and surrounding breast tissue. It may also involve removal of the entire breast and the muscle and lymph nodes below the breast if the cancer has begun to spread. This treatment is psychologically difficult for many women because it is disfiguring. Psychological support is especially necessary. Breast prostheses may also be helpful, but recent advances in breast reconstruction offer hope for those who must undergo this surgery.

DIAGNOSTIC AND TREATMENT PROCEDURES

The Pap smear, pelvic examination, laparoscopy, colposcopy, D&C, hysterectomy, and mammography have all been mentioned as procedures to diagnose and treat disorders and diseases of the female reproductive system. Since they are commonly used, each deserves more detailed description.

Pap Smear

The first step in the test is done by the physician, who uses a wooden spatula or pipette to take a cell sample from the patient's cervix and vagina. The specimen is smeared onto a slide and fixed with a fixing solution. The slide is then sent to a pathology laboratory for evaluation. The results are reported as follows:

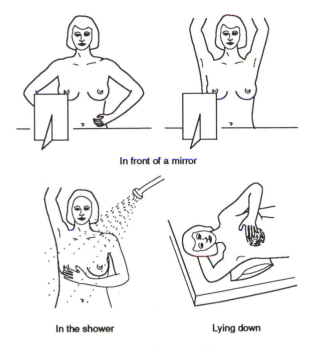

In front of a mirror

In the shower   Lying down

Figure 28: Positions for breast self-examination.

Class I - negative
Class II - abnormal but not malignant
Class III - suspicious
Class IV or V - probably malignant

Like any other test, the Pap smear is not always accurate. False-negative and false-positive results sometimes occur. Most physicians will investigate any abnormal Pap smear result with a follow-up examination and a biopsy. The test is a relatively inexpensive and accurate screening tool for cervical cancer.

Annual Pap smears are suggested for all women who are sexually active. All women should have a Pap smear by age 18. The American Cancer Society suggests that three consecutive normal smears should be obtained. After this, the test may be performed less frequently, but this is at the physician's discretion. Women who are at high risk for cancer or who have had positive test results should have Pap smears more often than others.

Pelvic Examination

The pelvic examination is a specific physical examination of the female reproductive system. In this procedure, the physician uses palpation (touch) and observation to determine the status of the reproductive organs. A trained physician can use his or her sense of touch to determine the location, shape, and mobility of the organs, and to detect growths or swellings.

The patient is placed in the dorsal recumbent or lithotomy position, on her back with her knees bent and her feet in stirrups. (See the book on clinical processes for a more detailed explanation of examination positions.) An instrument called a **speculum (SPECK yoo lum)** is used in the first step of a pelvic examination to widen the opening into the vagina. The physician inserts the speculum into the vaginal opening and focuses a light into the interior of the vagina. It is possible to visually examine the cervix and parts of the vaginal walls in this way.

The speculum is then removed. The physician puts on a sterile glove and inserts one or two fingers of one hand into the vagina. With the other hand, he or she palpates the outside of the abdomen. By skillful manipulation with both hands, the physician can determine the position and shape of the uterus and ovaries (see Figure 29). The examination may also include palpation through the rectum. A routine pelvic examination is usually combined with an annual examination of the breasts to detect new lumps or other abnormalities.

Mammography

A mammography (**mam OG rah fee**) is radiographic examination of breast tissue. It is a useful screening device for detecting breast malignancy, evaluating palpable and nonpalpable lumps, and differentiating between benign and cancerous breast diseases.

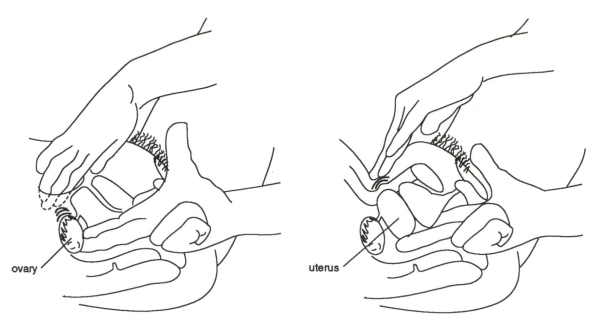

ovary

uterus

Figure 29: Bimanual pelvic examination.

The mammogram is done by having the patient rest one breast on a small examination table and compress it. Films from above, below, and the side are taken of each breast. Some patients find the procedure uncomfortable. It is recommended that women with no signs or history of breast cancer begin having mammograms at age 40. Mammograms should then be done every other year. An annual clinical breast examination is suggested yearly. From age 50 on, an annual clinical breast examination and mammogram should be performed. The American College of Obstetricians and Gynecologists further recommends a baseline mammogram between ages 35 and 39. Although mammography has a high false-positive rate, it has proven to be a reliable screening device.

Laparoscopy

Laparoscopy is a surgical technique that allows the physician to view the inside of the abdominal cavity. A laparoscope is used in the procedure. It is a long tube having a light and lens system so that an interior space can be seen and photographed.

The patient is given a general anesthetic. The laparoscope is then inserted through a small incision near the navel. The ovaries, uterine tubes, outside of the uterus, and other pelvic structures can thus be viewed. The laparoscope can also be used to remove small growths and tissue samples, with an attachment that has a claw-like instrument at one end. This tool can be introduced through the tube of the laparoscope and guided to the site of a growth or other abnormality with the optical system in the instrument. Sterilization can also be done using this technique, by burning the uterine tubes. (The procedure is commonly called "belly-button surgery.")

Colposcopy

A colposcope (a speculum with a magnifying lens) is used to visually examine the vagina and cervix.

Dilatation and Curettage (D&C)

The D&C is one of the most commonly performed gynecological procedures. General anesthesia is usually required. First, the cervix is dilated or opened by instruments called dilators. Once the cervix is opened, the physician can insert a curette into the uterus. The curette is a spoon-shaped instrument used to scrape material from the uterine walls and remove it. Sometimes removal of the material is the desired treatment. In other cases, the material is removed specifically for laboratory analysis.

Hysterectomy

Hysterectomy is the surgical removal of the uterus. The tubes and ovaries may be removed at the same time; this is called **bilateral salpingo oophorectomy (sal PING goh OH of oh RECK toh mee)**. It is included here not because it is performed in a medical office but because patients may have many questions and concerns about the procedure.

Hysterectomy is a controversial operation. Some critics charge that physicians have tended to perform the operation more often than necessary. However, there are many situations in which hysterectomy is either necessary or advisable.

A woman, especially a young one, who must have a hysterectomy may feel a strong sense of loss. She may fear that she will lose her womanhood. These fears are a normal reaction. However, many women have hysterectomies and continue to lead active and satisfying sex lives. If the ovaries are removed with the uterus, the patient's body will no longer secrete the hormones that the ovaries supplied. This can cause some of the uncomfortable physical and psychological symptoms of menopause. Replacement hormones may be prescribed in such cases to help ease these symptoms.

STOP AND REVIEW

Fill in the blanks.

1. One of the current treatments for premenstrual syndrome (PMS) is _____ _____.

2. Four organisms that can cause infections of the reproductive system are:

   a. _____

   b. _____

   c. _____

   d. _____

3. Two possible sources of these organisms are _____ and _____.

4. *Trichomonas* is a _____ organism and *Candida* is a _____ organism.

   a. bacterial

   b. fungal or yeast

   c. virus

   d. parasitic

5. The normal flora of the vagina reproduce too rapidly when the _____ balance of the vagina is upset.

6. _____ is infection of the breast.

7. Three symptoms of vaginitis are:

   a. _____

   b. _____

   c. _____

8. Blockages in the uterine tubes can be found by a test called the _____.

9. A ruptured ovarian cyst can cause peritonitis, or infection in the _____.

10. An instrument used to examine the ovary is called a _____.

11. Fibroids or myomas are benign tumors of the _____.

12. A common screening test to look for abnormal cells of cervical dysplasia is the _____.

13. The abnormal cells of the cervix may be cancerous and may be removed by:

    a. _____

    b. _____

    c. _____

(continued next page)

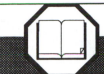

14. Cervical polyps are made of _____ tissue and can cause a _____ discharge.

15. The two most common cancers of the female reproductive system are _____ and _____.

16. _____ therapy usually follows surgical removal of cancerous tissue.

17. Name two instruments used to examine the female reproductive organs.

    a. _____

    b. _____

18. _____ is a sexually transmitted disease that can have serious consequences for a newborn.

19. _____ is a fatal STD that is becoming more common in women.

Short answers

20. What other parts or areas of the body are affected by a gonorrheal infection if it is not treated?

21. The first symptoms of syphilis are _____
    _____.

22. The treatment for syphilis is _____.

23. The final symptoms of syphilis include _____
    _____.

24. Herpes cannot be treated with antibiotics because _____
    _____.

25. Endometriosis is an abnormal growth of endometrial tissue which most commonly occurs _____.

26. Two methods of determining when ovulation occurs are _____
    _____.

27. Explain the differences between benign and malignant growths. _____
    _____

28. Explain the differences between a cyst and fibroadenoma. _____
    _____

29. Explain why ovarian cancer is difficult to detect. _____
    _____

30. Explain why breast cancer is a particularly dangerous form of cancer. _____
    _____

(continued next page)

31. A severe systemic infection that can occur during menstruation is _____.

32. Early detection of changes in the breast is done by a test called a_____.

33. Three benign breast tumors are:

a. _____

b. _____

c. _____

34. One type of uterine displacement is _____

_____

35. Match the following:

a. surgical removal of fibroids

b. x-ray test in which dye is inserted into the reproductive system

c. x-ray examination of the breasts

d. removal of the external female reproductive organs

e. excision of the breast

f. introduction of a scope into the vagina and cervix

g. surgical removal of the uterus

_____ 1. hysterectomy

_____ 2. colposcopy

_____ 3. vulvectomy

_____ 4. mastectomy

_____ 5. hysterosalpingography

_____ 6. myomectomy

_____ 7. mammography

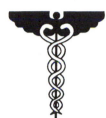

Knowledge Objectives

After completing this chapter you should be able to:

- define the terms pregnancy, embryo, and fetus
- name and describe two methods of estimating the due date of the newborn
- list the seven early signs of pregnancy
- describe the process of fertilization from ovulation to zygote formation and then to embryo development
- identify the optimum time for fertilization
- describe how chromosomes determine sex
- describe the function of the placenta
- name and describe the three stages of development during pregnancy
- describe the differences between a full-term and a premature infant
- describe three methods of monitoring fetal growth
- describe the changes in a pregnant woman's body and their causes
- describe three events that signal the beginning of childbirth
- name and describe the stages of labor
- explain how the breasts produce milk
- define Apgar score and explain how it is used
- name some common congenital defects
- list the tests, measurements, and examinations done during prenatal care
- list and describe seven complications of pregnancy
- explain how a maternal disease or infection can affect the fetus
- list and describe six complications of labor

Pregnancy, Parturition, and the Newborn

INTRODUCTION

The term **pregnancy (PREG nan see)** means having a developing embryo or fetus in the body as a result of the union of a sperm and an ovum. The term **parturition (PAR tyoo RISH un)** refers to the labor and delivery period. This chapter will cover pregnancy and parturition, and briefly will address the newborn.

On the average, the full development of a human being requires 280 days or 40 weeks, but the time period varies. A full-term pregnancy is one in which the fetus has remained in the womb for the entire time necessary for development. A **premature delivery** is one in which the infant is born before term, or before it is fully mature and ready for birth. Another common term used in discussions of pregnancy is **gestation (jes TAY shun)**, which means the period of time during which the embryo or fetus has been developing since the ovum was fertilized.

Determining the due date, or the approximate date the infant will be born, is still an inexact science. It is impossible to know exactly when the ovum and sperm were united, because of the variation in ovarian cycles and the possibility that sperm can live for several days after intercourse. The date is usually estimated in one of two ways—by counting forward 40 weeks from the woman's last menstrual period, or by using **Nagele's (NAY geh leez) rule**.

In Nagele's rule, the estimated date of confinement or delivery (EDC or EDD) is determined by counting back 3 months from the first day of the last period, then adding 7 days. This date, then, in the following year, will be the EDC. Both of these methods are based on the assumption that ovulation occurs 14 days after the last period, but this is not always the case. Also, some women have slight bleeding in the first month of pregnancy, which can be mistaken for a normal period. For these reasons, the delivery date may have to be revised several times as the physician observes changes in the pregnant woman's body and in the developing fetus or embryo. As the pregnancy progresses, ultrasonography may provide a more accurate estimate of fetal age and EDC.

DIAGNOSIS OF PREGNANCY

A number of outward signs occur early in

pregnancy. To confirm a diagnosis, blood and/or urine tests are done. The early signs include:

1. Absence of Menstrual Periods. After an ovum has been fertilized, the corpus luteum in the ovary produces the hormone progesterone. At the same time, the egg-production function of both ovaries is suspended until the pregnancy is completed or terminated. Therefore, the lining of the uterus is maintained rather than shed, and menstruation does not occur.

2. Nausea and Vomiting. Nausea occurs in about 50 percent of pregnant women. Vomiting occurs in about 33 percent. It is not known exactly what causes these indications of pregnancy, but they may result from high estrogen levels in the bloodstream. In most cases, they occur early in pregnancy and disappear by the end of the third month.

3. Abnormally Frequent Urination. The reason for frequent urination early in pregnancy is not fully understood, but generally it results from changes in the urinary tract, including an increase in blood plasma filtration in the kidney and a shift in the position of the uterus in relation to the ureters and bladder.

4. Increased Breast Tenderness and Breast Enlargement. This sign occurs because of the development of additional milk ducts in the breasts and also increased fat deposits in the breasts. These changes may cause tingling, tenderness, or even pain.

5. Darkening of the Nipples and Areola. The cause of this darkening is not known, but the change is usually permanent in fair-skinned women.

6. Thickening of Vagina and Development of Purplish Color in Vagina and Cervix (Chadwick's Sign). Changes in the vagina make it increasingly stretchable as term approaches, to allow the fetus to pass through it during childbirth. This process begins in the first weeks of pregnancy. The vagina becomes a dusky color instead of the normal pink, and the vaginal walls thicken. The vagina is especially susceptible to infection during pregnancy because of these and other changes.

7. Softening of the Cervix (Goodell's sign.) About 5 to 6 weeks after fertilization, the cervix becomes softer. This probably is caused by an increase in blood vessel penetration to the cervix. The cervix remains in this condition until a few weeks before delivery, when it begins to open to allow the fetus to emerge from the uterus.

When some or all of these signs are present, and especially when a woman who usually has regular menstruation has missed two successive periods, a pregnancy test is done. Blood or urine is tested for human chorionic gonadotropin (HCG) described earlier. This hormone is secreted by cells surrounding the fertilized egg and by the placenta which develops from these cells. HCG can be detected with a blood test even before the first missed period.

FERTILIZATION

At ovulation, a mature ovum is released by an ovarian follicle and normally is pulled from the ovary into the uterine tube. The ovum then travels along the tube toward the uterus. It remains alive and fertilizable for 14 to 24 hours after it is released by the ovary. At the same time, changes occur in the cervical mucus that create a favorable environment for sperm movement through the cervix to the uterus.

The sperm are ejaculated through the male penis, which is inserted into the female vagina during sexual intercourse. Normally, 2 to 5 ml of semen containing about 70 million sperm per milliliter (or between 140 and 350 million sperm) are deposited in the vagina. About 75 percent of the sperm are normal, and about half of those are motile. If conditions are favorable for fertilization, perhaps 50 or fewer of the motile sperm will make their way through the uterus to a uterine tube in the next hour. These sperm may make contact with an ovum. Sperm usually survive for 24 to 72 hours, though they may survive for up to 6 days.

The optimal time for fertilization is not more than 72 hours before ovulation and not more than 24 hours after ovulation. A couple who wishes to have a child can use the same basic technique for calculating ovulation as a couple who use the rhythm method to prevent conception. Based on the woman's usual cycle and on changes in her body temperature, the date of ovulation can be estimated. Ovulation usually occurs on Day 14, 15, or 16 of the menstrual cycle. To promote conception, the couple should have intercourse as close to the time of ovulation as possible.

Once sperm and ovum come together, usually in the section of the uterine tube closest to the ovary, the sperm attempt to penetrate the ovum. The ovum is surrounded by a tough membrane called the **zona pellucida (ZOH nah peh LOO sih duh),** which the sperm must penetrate to fertilize the ovum. This process is aided by enzymes produced by the sperm. Once one sperm penetrates the zona pellucida, the

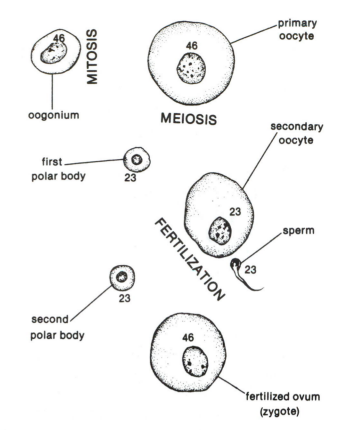

Figure 30: Oogenesis and fertilization. Mitosis of a primordial egg cell (oogonium) present in the ovary since birth produces a primary oocyte with 46 chromosomes. Through meiosis, this oocyte produces a secondary oocyte with 23 chromosomes, a smaller polar body containing the other 23. At ovulation, the secondary oocyte is not fully mature. If fertilized, it again divides unequally, producing another polar body and a fertilized ovum (zygote) containing 46 chromosomes and most of the cytoplasm. The polar bodies disintegrate.

membrane becomes impenetrable.

When the sperm enters the ovum, its tail drops off and its head unites with the nucleus of the ovum. Together, they form a **zygote (ZY got)** (see Figure 30). The ovum and sperm each have 23 chromosomes. Together they have 46 chromosomes, the number necessary to make a human being.

The sex of the embryo is determined at this point. The ovum has 22 autosomal chro-

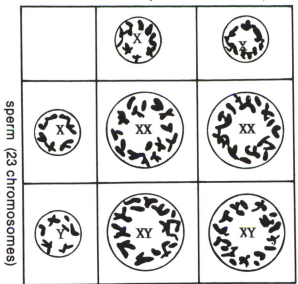

ova (23 chromosomes)

sperm (23 chromosomes)

Four possible
46-chromosome zygotes

Figure 31: Sex determination. Meiosis of a male cell produces two sperm, one carrying an X-chromosome and one carrying a Y. Meiosis of a female cell produces two ova, both carrying X-chromosomes. Possible offspring can then be male (XY) or female (XX) in one of four combinations.

mosomes, and one X-chromosome. The sperm has 22 autosomes, and an X- or a Y-chromosome. If the sperm has a X-chromosome, the offspring will be female; if it has a Y-chromosome, the offspring will be male (see Figure 31).

The single, united cell then begins to multiply by **mitosis (my TOH sis),** creating more and more cells that have the same genetic makeup as the zygote. As the cells reproduce, the ball of cells moves toward the uterus (see Figure 32).

At first, the ball is solid. In this stage, it is called a **morula (MOR yoo lah).** About the fifth day, the morula begins to change to a hollow, fluid-filled

ball called a **blastocyst (BLAS toh sist).** About the sixth day, the ball reaches the uterus and floats freely for about another day. By halfway through the seventh day after conception, the ball usually becomes implanted in the lining of the uterus. At this point, the blastocyst has an outer wall of cells called **trophoblast (TROF oh blast)** cells, a cell mass attached to the inner surface of the ball, and a filling of fluid. The inner mass becomes the **embryo (EM bree oh);** the trophoblast cells become parts of the **placenta (plah SEN tah),** the **amnion (AM nee on), chorion (KOH ree on),** and **yolk sac** (see Figure 33).

The chorion and amnion are membranes that surround the embryo. The chorion is the outer layer, which is closer to the maternal tissue. Through this membrane, the exchange of oxygen, nutrients, and waste materials between mother and fetus occurs

THE DEVELOPMENT OF TWINS

In order for identical twins to develop, the zygote has one additional division and then splits apart, producing two separate but almost identical zygotes. Two fetuses of the same sex develop from one egg and one sperm, usually share one placenta and chorion, but have separate amnions. There seems to be no hereditary factor for identical twins.

Nonidentical (fraternal) twins occur when the mother produces two eggs during the same cycle, both of which are fertilized by different sperm. Fraternal twins can be the same sex or one male and one female. They always have separate placentas, amnions, and chorions. The tendency toward fraternal twins seems to be familial.

Age is a factor in producing twins. Women in their late thirties are more likely to produce two eggs during one cycle. Women who already have three or more children have the same tendency. Women who have been given drugs to induce ovulation also are more likely to have nonidentical twins or other multiple births.

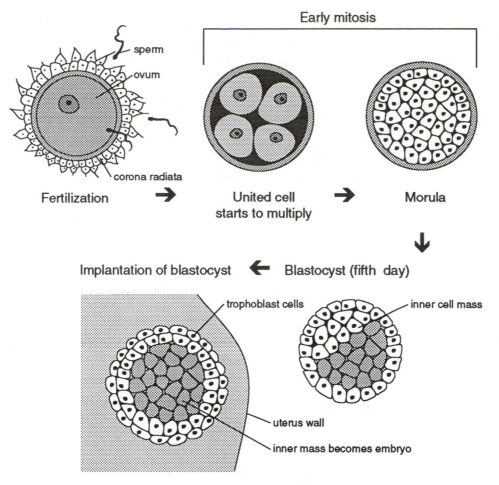

Figure 32: Fertilization, zygote, and blastocyst development, and implantation of blastocyst on uterine lining.

in the area of the placenta. The amnion is the inner membrane, closer to the fetus, which contains the amniotic fluid. This is the fluid in which the developing embryo or fetus floats until just before birth.

IMPLANTATION

During ovulation, fertilization, and the first cell divisions of the zygote, the lining of the uterus becomes thick and its blood vessels expand. These changes in the endometrium prepare it for implantation of the blastocyst. As the blastocyst enters the uterus, projections called **chorionic villi (koh ree AHN ick VIL iy)** develop in the chorion, and capillaries expand to reach the endometrium, bringing a supply of maternal blood close to

the surface of the uterine wall. The blastocyst then burrows into the endometrium, usually about halfway down the uterus. The surface of the uterine lining closes over the blastocyst, leaving only a small bulge on the surface.

FORMATION OF PLACENTA

At this point, the placenta begins to form from trophoblast cells and maternal cells. At the same time, the corpus luteum in the ovary secretes the hormones progesterone and estrogen to maintain the uterine lining so that the implanted embryo can remain in the uterus. If the corpus luteum should disappear, as it does when the ovum released by the ovary is not fertilized, the uterine lin-

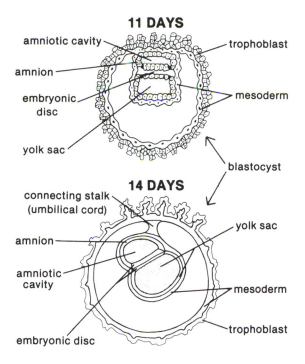

11 DAYS

amniotic cavity — trophoblast
amnion
embryonic disc — mesoderm
yolk sac
blastocyst

14 DAYS

connecting stalk (umbilical cord)
amnion — yolk sac
amniotic cavity — mesoderm
embryonic disc — trophoblast

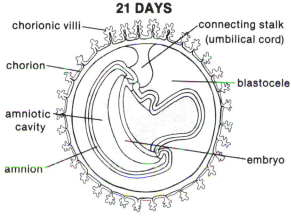

21 DAYS

chorionic villi — connecting stalk (umbilical cord)
chorion — blastocele
amniotic cavity — embryo
amnion

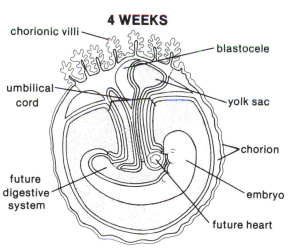

4 WEEKS

chorionic villi — blastocele
umbilical cord — yolk sac
future digestive system — chorion
— embryo
future heart

Figure 33: Stages in fetal development, from 11 days to 4 weeks.

ing would be shed in a normal menstrual period.

UMBILICAL CORD

The placenta develops fully by the third month of pregnancy, then continues to grow with the fetus until term. The placenta forms on the uterine wall, usually where the maternal blood supply is the best. It is joined to the fetus by the **umbilical (um BIL ih kal) cord.** The placenta is made up of connective tissue and endothelial tissue that support a network of blood vessels. The maternal surface is convoluted by villi, or finger-like projections, that are anchored to similar projections in the uterine lining (the chorionic villi). On both sides are blood vessels, separated by the chorionic membrane. The placental vessels contain fetal blood, and the uterine vessels hold maternal blood. Exchange of oxygen, carbon dioxide, nutrients, and waste materials occurs across the chorion, without mixing of maternal and fetal blood. The fetal side of the placenta is smooth except where the umbilical cord enters. The umbilical cord usually has one vein and two arteries, which convey fetal blood back and forth to the placenta.

This connection via the placenta continues throughout fetal development, until the umbilical cord is severed at birth. However, the placenta does begin to decrease in efficiency at the end of pregnancy, especially if delivery is delayed past term.

The placenta also functions as a temporary endocrine gland. It secretes HCG early in pregnancy, as it develops. This hormone stimulates the corpus luteum, which produces progesterone and estrogen to maintain the uterine lining. The amount of HCG peaks at about the sixtieth to the seventieth day of gestation and then gradually declines. The corpus luteum then gradually disap-

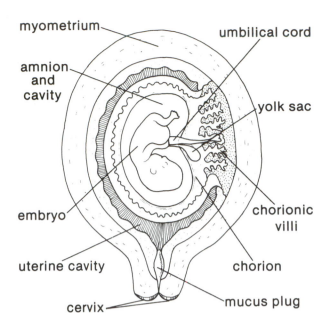

myometrium

amnion and cavity

umbilical cord

yolk sac

embryo

chorionic villi

uterine cavity

chorion

cervix

mucus plug

Figure 34: Embryo at 8 weeks.

pears, and the placenta takes over production of progesterone and estrogen.

EMBRYONIC AND FETAL DEVELOPMENT

A developing infant is considered an embryo from the time of implantation of the blastocyst in the uterine wall in the second week of gestation through the eighth week of development. Thereafter, it is usually called a **fetus (FEE tus)**. Some experts make this division at the eleventh week, because all the organs are present at that time and development enters a new stage. Figure 33 shows the embryo at the eleventh, fourteenth, twenty-first, and twenty-eighth days of development. Figure 34 shows the embryo at 8 weeks (56 days).

First Trimester

The first stage of development is often called the first trimester of pregnancy. It is also called differentiation. During the first 8-week period, the blastocyst is implanted, the amnion, chorion, and placenta form, the yolk sac disappears, and the major internal and external structures are formed. All the different types of cells found in the human are differentiated from each other.

During this time, the embryo is very susceptible to **teratogens (TER ah toh jens)**, agents or factors that cause defects. This is because organs and structures are most likely to be damaged as they develop. Once they are present, they are far less likely to be affected. By the end of 8 weeks, the embryo is about 2.5 cm long and weighs about 4 gm.

By the end of the third month, the organ systems are fully formed (though not mature). The embryo, now a fetus, can move its limbs. It can make sucking motions and change its facial expression. At this point, the fetus weighs about 5 gm and is about 9 cm long.

Second Trimester

The next period of development is called the second trimester. It is a period of rapid growth. In the fourth month, the fetus grows considerably, from about 9 cm to 14 cm long, and from 5 gm to 115 gm. Also, the bones begin to harden or ossify.

In the fifth month, the fetus begins to develop hair and to move in the uterus. Its heartbeat is 120 to 160 beats per minute. It has grown to 30 cm in length and weighs about 300 gm. However, the fetus probably could not yet survive outside the mother's body.

Starting with the sixth month of pregnancy, the fetus's chances of survival outside the mother gradually increase. The fetus more than doubles in weight during this 4-week period, to about 650 gm, and it grows about 4 cm. The organs and body structures continue to mature.

Third Trimester

The final period of pregnancy, the third trimester, is a time when the mother's intake of protein is especially important. The fetus is producing brain cells at a rapid rate in the seventh and eighth months. It also more than doubles in weight, to about 2,000 gm, and grows about 10 cm. In the ninth month, growth slows somewhat and final maturing processes occur. Among the last organs to mature are the lungs because they are not used by the fetus until birth. A normal full-term infant weighs approximately 3,300 to 3,600 gm at birth, or 6 lbs. 14 oz. to 7 lbs. 8 oz. Of course, normal infants may weigh more or less than this. An immature or premature infant is defined as one weighing less than 2,500 gm (5 lbs. 8 oz.) at birth. See Table 6 for a summary of fetal development.

MONITORING FETAL WELL-BEING

The progress of fetal well-being and development can be followed with several different medical procedures including ultrasound scans, **amniocentesis (AM nee oh sen TEE sis),** the biophysical profile, monitoring of the fetal heart rate, the nonstress test, fetal movement count, and chorionic villus sampling.

Ultrasound Scans

Ultrasound, or ultrasonography, is a method of creating an image of the fetus using sound waves. It is considerably safer for the fetus than the use of x-rays for the same purpose.

Table 6: Timetable of Human Fetal Development

Week(s)	Development
1	Fertilization and implantation.
2	Placental circulation begins in primitive form.
3	Period missed. Cardiovasular system begins to develop.
4	Fetal heart begins to beat. Arm and leg buds appear.
5–8	All essential structures develop in primitive form. Week 8 last week of embryonic period.
9–10	Fetal period begins. Face begins to look human, genitalia have male or female characteristics, but not completely formed.
11–12	Sex distinguishable. Body length doubles. Head is half of body length. All organs are present.
13–16	Rapid growth. Ossification of skeleton progresses. Head smaller relative to rest of body.
17–20	Fetal movements felt by mother (quickening). Normal body proportions reached. Fine hair all over skin.
21–25	Weight gain. All organs well developed except respiratory system.
26–29	Survival outside mother's body possible but still difficult. Head hair developed, fat layers under skin begin to form.
30–34	Fat deposits increase. Skin smooth, limbs look chubby.
35–38	Finishing period. Growth slows. Fat deposits increase. Head has largest circumference of all body parts. Lungs develop completely.

Source: Moore, Keith L., *The Developing Human: Clinically Oriented Embryology* (2nd Edition), W.B. Saunders, Philadelphia, 1977, pp. 2–5, 81–91.

This technique is used mostly to determine the size and position of the fetus. It also is often used as a preliminary step in amniocentesis.

Amniocentesis

In amniocentesis, a needle is inserted into the amniotic sac to remove a sample of amniotic fluid. It is important in this procedure to avoid inserting the needle into the fetus or the umbilical cord, so ultrasound is done first to locate the fetus. The amniotic fluid can be analyzed to determine if there are certain genetic abnormalities in the fetus such as Down's syndrome, or whether the fetus is mature and can be delivered safely.

Biophysical Profile

Sometimes a biophysical profile using ultrasonography may be done. The fetus and amniotic sac are visualized using ultrasound. Fetal breathing, gross body movement, fetal muscle tone, and amniotic fluid volume are evaluated. A biophysical score is assigned. The highest possible score is 8. A score of 6 indicates a need to perform the nonstress test in 24 hours. A score of 4 necessitates immediate delivery by induction of labor or cesarean section.

Monitoring of the Fetal Heart Rate

Monitoring of the fetal heart rate can be done indirectly before labor begins, by attaching a sensor to the mother's abdomen. After labor begins and the membranes that surround the fetus have broken, fetal heartbeat can be monitored directly by placing sensors on the fetus. Delivery is a particularly crucial time for such monitoring, because the fetus is under considerable stress as it passes through the birth canal. If the fetus is in difficulty, fetal monitoring can detect the problem and the obstetrician can often take steps to prevent fetal damage and ensure a healthy delivery.

Nonstress Test (NST)

The nonstress test is a noninvasive test done to assess fetal well-being. The test is done in a physician's office or in a hospital outpatient facility by a nurse and requires 20 to 30 minutes or more to complete depending on the activity level of the fetus. NSTs are used in high-risk pregnancy conditions, including postdate pregnancy, a small-for-gestational-age fetus, decreased fetal movement, maternal diabetes, preeclampsia, or other maternal medical conditions. The test is usually done in the third trimester and measures the response of the fetal heart to fetal movement.

Absent or limited fetal activity or heart rate acceleration in response to movement results in a nonreactive NST and indicates the need for further testing and possible delivery by induction of labor. An NST with adequate fetal movement and heart rate accelerations is a reactive NST. The test is done by placing an ultrasound sensor on the mother's abdomen. The sensor transmits the fetal heart tone to a monitor, which prints out a tracing or monitor strip. The strip is then reviewed by the physician and diagnosed as reactive or nonreactive.

Fetal Movement Count

Fetal movement count is done by the mother at home. She counts the number of fetal movements in a 30-minute period three times a day. Decreased fetal movement may indicate the need for an NST.

Chorionic Villus Sampling (CVS)

Unlike the previously discussed tests, CVS is an invasive procedure which evaluates the fetus for genetic disorders. CVS, however, is done in the first trimester (as early as 5 weeks), earlier than amniocentesis. This allows for an earlier and safer abortion option if genetic defects are present.

The fetal sac and placenta are visualized by ultrasound. A small catheter is inserted through the cervix, and a portion of chorion is aspirated. Complications of this procedure include spontaneous abortion, infection, hematoma, intrauterine growth retardation, and trauma.

EFFECTS OF PREGNANCY ON THE MOTHER

As the embryo, then the fetus, develops in her uterus, the mother's body naturally undergoes a number of changes. Some of these changes probably are caused by the different levels of hormones required to produce a human being. Others occur because of the change in weight and balance caused by the growing fetus in the uterus. Still other changes prepare the pregnant woman's body for labor and delivery.

For example, the ligaments that hold the joints of the skeleton together become slightly more elastic, so that the pelvis can expand during childbirth to allow passage through the pelvic opening. An effect of this change is the back pain associated with pregnancy. The back is especially vulnerable because of the strain involved in carrying the extra weight.

Other bodily and emotional changes in pregnant women are not well understood. For example, the feeling of well-being, and sometimes even euphoria, that many women have during the second trimester of pregnancy has not been explained. Also, the loss of coordination that usually occurs during pregnancy has not yet been traced to any particular cause.

A pregnant woman has special needs. For example, during the first trimester of pregnancy many women feel very tired and need extra sleep. Also, the pregnant woman needs to be particularly careful to eat a bal-

anced, nutritious diet. Often a woman will have cravings for foods she normally would not eat, or aversions to foods she normally would enjoy. For example, many women develop an aversion to alcohol during pregnancy.

Table 7 lists some of the changes that occur in normal pregnancy and their causes (if known). Many subtle changes in body chemistry and structure also occur. Most of these features of pregnancy disappear within a few weeks of delivery.

PRENATAL CARE

Certain screening tests are a normal part of prenatal care. These include blood pressure measurement, urinalysis, and blood tests. High blood pressure can cause serious complications in the later stages of pregnancy, so the blood pressure is monitored throughout. Urinalysis is done to determine whether the patient has diabetes mellitus or an asymptomatic bladder infection. Some women develop diabetes during pregnancy, and this can affect normal fetal development. The mother's blood type is determined to assess the possibility of incompatibility between blood types in the mother and fetus. Blood tests are also done to detect immunity to German measles, signs of STDs, and indications of anemia.

Assessment of these factors and also the age and history of the patient enable the physician to classify each pregnant woman as high-risk or low-risk. Of course, this initial assessment can change if new developments occur during the pregnancy. The assessment determines how often the patient needs to be seen by the physician and how closely certain aspects of fetal development and maternal health must be monitored.

During prenatal visits, the woman can discuss common pregnancy problems, such

Table 7: Changes in Maternal Physiology During Pregnancy

System	Change	Cause
Central Nervous System	1sts trimester: fatigue, extra sleep, nausea, vomiting 2nd trimester: duphoria 3rd trimester: depressuin, fatigue coordination reduced	Possibly high progesterone levels
Respiratory System	Elevation of diaphragam Increased tidal volume (hyperventilation of pregnancy)	Growth of fetus in uterus High progresterone levels
Cardiovascular System	Heart pushed up and to the left Decreased blood pressure (until late in pregnancy) Increased cardiac output blood vessels dilate and composition of walls changes	Elevation of diaphragm Unknown Possibly high estrogen levels Unknown
Blood	Increase in volume Increase in number of blood cells, platelets Chemical changes	Possibly increased aldosterone and estrogen Increased respiration (tidal volume), high estrogen levels
Gastrointestinal System	Acid reflux (heartburn) Constipation	Loss of smooth muscle tone Slowing muscle action in digestive tract
Urinary Tract	Increased kidney activity Frequent urination	Unknown Compression of bladder by fetus
Skin	Changes in pigmentation: face areola of breasts Stretch marks	Increase in deposits of pigment Distention of abdomen
General	Increases storage of fat Increased storage of minreals Enlargement of breasts	Unknown Storage mainly in fetus Growth of milk ducts

as leg cramps, constipation, and heartburn, and learn how to manage them. In prenatal classes, prospective parents can learn about labor, delivery, and child care. The physician may refer patients to these classes.

LABOR AND DELIVERY

A technical term often used for the process of labor and delivery is parturition. The process is extremely variable, so a brief description of it necessarily covers only the usual order and timing of events. Remember that there are many exceptions, depending on the individual woman's physical characteristics, the position of the fetus, and whether or not the woman has had children before, to name just a few of the influential factors.

Parturition starts a few weeks before labor begins, with three events. The fetus settles into the pelvic area 2 to 4 weeks before the onset of labor. This is called **lightening**.

Also, a type of irregular contraction called a **Braxton-Hicks contraction** occurs with increasing frequency in the final month before labor. In women who have not previously given birth, these contractions of the uterine muscle usually are not painful until about 1 hour before labor begins. In women who have previously had several children, Braxton-Hicks contractions may cause discomfort or pain as early as the fifth month of pregnancy.

Finally, the cervix becomes softer and thinner, in a process called cervical **effacement (eh FAYS ment),** starting about 1

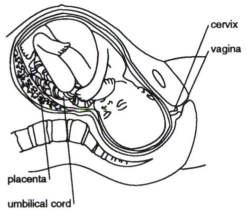

cervix
vagina
placenta
umbilical cord

Fully developed fetus

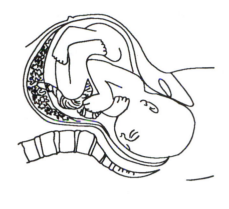

Dilation stage

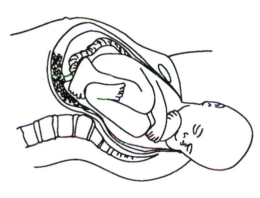

Expulsion stage

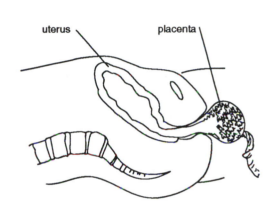

uterus   placenta

Placental stage

Figure 35: Three stages of labor.

month before delivery.

There are three stages of labor (see Figure 35) that vary in length and difficulty from patient to patient. Generally, a woman's first experience is longer than later ones.

The First Stage

The first stage of labor is the dilation stage (see Figure 35). The purpose of this stage is to open the cervix. Throughout pregnancy, the cervix maintains the fetus inside the uterus. At the end of pregnancy, this structure must enlarge to allow delivery of the fully developed fetus. The process of change begins with effacement, then continues as

labor begins. Usually one of the first signs of labor is expulsion of a plug of mucus that forms in the cervical opening early in pregnancy. The appearance of this plug, which is a small piece of bloody tissue, is called the show. Another sign that labor is starting is the breaking of the amnionic sac and discharge of the fluid that surrounded the fetus. This is called breaking water.

The first stage of labor may be divided into three phases: latent (with cervical dilation up to 4 cm), active (with dilation from 5 to 7 cm), and transition (with dilation from 8 to 10 cm). The mechanism for dilation of the cervix is contractions of the muscular uterine walls. Unlike Braxton-Hicks contractions, which are irregular and uncoordinated, labor contractions are regular and smooth. At first they occur 15 to 20 minutes apart, but they gradually come closer together until they occur 1 to 2 minutes apart. In a first pregnancy, this stage lasts on average 12 hours. In later births, it usually requires 4 to 8 hours. At the end of the first stage of labor, the cervix is completely effaced—it has disappeared into the wall of the uterus. The opening between the uterus and the vagina is about 10 cm in diameter, and the head is protruding (if the fetus is in the normal position for delivery).

The Second Stage

The second stage of labor is the expulsion stage (see Figure 35). Contractions are powerful and last from 50 to 90 seconds. They include an urge to bear down, which serves to push the fetus out the birth canal. This stage lasts until the infant emerges completely from the canal. This requires about 1 hour for a first birth and less for later ones.

At this point, the umbilical cord can be cut, separating the infant from the placenta.

The Third Stage

This stage of labor is necessary to expel the placenta from the uterus and return the uterus to its normal (nonpregnant) size and shape. This stage is therefore called the **placental stage** (see Figure 35). The uterus must continue to contract even after the placenta emerges, to prevent excessive bleeding from the blood vessels that fed the fetus through the placenta and umbilical cord.

The third stage of labor usually requires about 15 minutes. All three stages combined may consume a full 24-hour day to less than 5 hours.

With the birth of the baby, the pregnancy is ended and the mother enters the **postpartal** period.

THE POSTPARTAL PERIOD

In the weeks and months after delivery, the mother's body undergoes many physical changes. However, if she plans to breastfeed the infant, her breasts will not return to the pre-pregnant state until after she discontinues breastfeeding. During the postpartal period, the woman also may experience psychological or emotional changes.

Physical Changes

The decrease in estrogen and progesterone levels after delivery stimulates the reversal of many pregnancy-induced changes. Within 6 weeks after delivery, the uterus undergoes **involution (IN voh LOO shun),** a process that returns it nearly to its pre-pregnancy size and shape. The uterus also sloughs off its lining, producing **lochia (LOH kee ah;** uterine discharge) in three stages. Lochia alba is a bloody discharge with a fleshy odor that lasts 1 to 4 days postpartum. Lochia serosa is pinkish-brown and odorless and occurs 5 to 7 days postpartum. Lochia alba may be cream-colored or colorless and may smell slightly stale. It occurs from 1 to 3 weeks postpartum.

In a woman who does not breastfeed, menstruation usually resumes in 7 to 9 weeks after childbirth. In a woman who breastfeeds, menstruation occurs later.

Pregnancy-induced changes in other body systems usually reverse naturally. However, weakened breast and abdominal muscles may require exercise to return them to normal.

Lactation

By the end of pregnancy, the breasts have developed sufficiently to engage in **lactation (lack TAY shun;** milk secretion). They contain a fluid called **colostrum (kuh LOS trum),** which has all the components of

Table 8: Scale for Apgar Rating

	0	1	2
Appearance (skin color)	White or blue	Limbs blue, body pink	Pink
Pulse (rate)	No pulse	100 beats/min	>100 beats/min
Grimace (reflexive grimace initiated by stimulating the plantar surface of the foot)	No response	Facial grimaces, slight body movement	Facial grimaces, extensive body movement
Activity (muscle tone)	No movement, muscles flaccid	Limbs partially flexed, little movement, poor muscle tone	Active movement, good muscle tone
Respiratory effort (amount of respiratory activity)	No respiration	Slow, irregular respiration	Good, regular respiration, strong cry

breast milk except fat. The fat accumulates in the 2 to 4 days immediately after delivery. There are two hormones, **oxytocin (OCK seh TOH sin)** and **prolactin (proh LACK tin),** involved in milk production. Oxytocin is stored in the posterior lobe of the pituitary gland. In response to the infant's sucking on the breasts, this hormone is released into the bloodstream. It stimulates the milk-producing glands to contract and eject milk into the milk ducts. Prolactin is produced by the anterior pituitary gland at the same time, to sustain milk production. When the original stimulus of sucking is removed, the breasts gradually stop producing milk.

Psychological Changes

The rapid reversal of physical changes shortly after birth, coupled with the physical stress of labor and delivery, can leave a new mother exhausted and sometimes depressed. The added stress of taking care of a totally dependent infant makes the first few weeks and months of parenthood very difficult physically and emotionally. Anyone who is working with new mothers should be aware of these difficulties and make a special effort to be helpful and supportive.

THE NEWBORN

Immediately after birth, the physician examines and tests the newborn to discover any apparent congenital defects and to evaluate its health. Usually the Apgar scoring system is used for the initial assessment. In this system five signs are checked and assigned a score of 0, 1, or 2. The signs are heart rate, respiratory rate, muscle tone, reflex irritability, and color (see Table 8). All of these signs can be quickly assessed. A perfectly normal child will have an Apgar score of 10 within 1 minute of birth. A score of 4 to 6 means that the newborn needs some assistance to establish breathing and other normal functions. If the score is 0 to 2, the newborn needs emergency treatment. Apgar scores are recorded at both 1 and 5 minutes after birth. The 5-minute score is the more accurate gauge of potential problems.

Congenital Defects

The physician also examines the newborn visually for defects, such as cleft palate, hip dislocation, and signs of Down's syndrome. Congenital defects may be genetic (inherited) or may be caused by teratogens. They

Table 9: Congenital Defects

Defect	Definition
Transposition of the great vessels	In the heart, the aorta and the pulmonary artery are reversed.
Atrial septal defect	A hole in an atrial wall of the heart
Ventricular septal defect	A hole in a ventricular wall of the heart
Congential pulmonic or aortic stenosis	Narrowing of the pulmonary artery or aorta
Patent ductus arteriosus	Extra blood vessel in fetal heart fails to close off at birth
Club foot (talipes)	Foot or feet bent in wrong direction
Dislocation of the hip	Hip joint out of place
Cleft lip	Vertical split in upper lip
Down's syndrome	Chromosomal abnormality that causes severe retardation
Spina bifida	Defect in spinal column
Phenylketonuria (PKU)	Genetic disorder in which an enzyme is missing from the body
Hydrocephalus	Fluid in the skull that causes the head to be abnormally large. Can lead to retardation if severe.

range from serious malformations that shorten the child's life or prevent normal development, to minor problems that can be corrected completely in the first weeks or months of life. Some congenital defects are apparent in the initial examination immediately after birth. Others may not be discovered until the child is more than 1 year old.

Table 9 lists a few common congenital problems of the newborn. The exact cause of many of these problems is not known, but some of them may be genetic disorders. Other defects are the result of environmental factors, including maternal illness during pregnancy, and drug use by the mother. Some examples are German measles contracted by the mother, especially in the first trimester of pregnancy, and the fetal alcohol syndrome. German measles is a minor viral infection in adults. However, the virus can cross the placenta to the embryo and cause serious abnormalities. In the first trimester of pregnancy especially, when cells are differentiating and organs are forming, heart defects and other major abnormalities can result from the infection.

Fetal alcohol syndrome is a group of signs and symptoms, such as a characteristic facial appearance and certain behavioral problems, that have been linked with heavy drinking by the mother during pregnancy.

Certain drugs can also cause abnormalities in the fetus if they are taken during pregnancy. For example, the drug diethylstilbestrol (DES) was used in the 1950s to prevent miscarriage, but was later found to cause susceptibility to reproductive tract cancer in female offspring. Also, thalidomide, which was prescribed in the 1960s as a sedative for pregnant women, mainly in Europe, caused severe limb defects in their offspring. In general, pregnant women are told by their physicians to avoid drugs of any kind, alcohol, and smoking to reduce the possibility of birth defects.

DISORDERS OF PREGNANCY AND PARTURITION

Parity and Gravida

Gravida is a term frequently used in the medical profession to describe a woman's pregnancy status. If it is her first pregnancy she is described as primigravida, secundigravida if in her second pregnancy, and so on, using the appropriate Latin numerical prefix. Parity is a descriptive word also commonly used in the obstetrician's office. If a woman has parity, she has given birth to an infant or infants, alive or dead.

Pregnancy Disorders

Most pregnancies proceed normally from conception to delivery, but sometimes complications occur. These may be caused by abnormalities in the mother or the fetus, or by diseases that occur during pregnancy. Prenatal care is an important factor in ensuring a healthy pregnancy and in preventing any problems that develop from becoming severe or life-threatening to the mother or the fetus.

Ectopic Pregnancy. In this condition, the fertilized egg is implanted outside the uterus. The most common implantation site in this disorder is the uterine tube. The blastocyst burrows into the wall of the tube and usually penetrates an artery, causing bleeding. The bleeding dislodges the embryo, usually within 14 days of fertilization. However, sometimes the pregnancy continues for several weeks, and eventually ruptures the uterine tube.

The usual symptoms of **ectopic (eck TOP ick) pregnancy** are abdominal pain and vaginal bleeding. The bleeding may be mistaken for menstrual bleeding unless it is extremely heavy, or it may be internal and not be apparent. Heavy vaginal or internal bleeding from ectopic pregnancy can lead to shock. If the uterine tube ruptures, or if the embryo is implanted in the abdominal cavity, severe infection may occur.

Diagnosis of ectopic pregnancy is usually made by ultrasound scan and laparoscopy. The scan may show the location of an abnormality in the abdominal area. The laparoscope allows the physician to view the abnormality to determine its nature. The treatment is immediate surgery to remove the embryo and placenta and repair the damage. The affected uterine tube may have to be removed.

Once a woman has had an ectopic pregnancy, the likelihood of her having another one is increased. However, normal pregnancy may be possible. Other factors that increase the risk of ectopic pregnancy are previous abortions, damage to or abnormality of the uterine tubes, use of an IUD for contraception, and previous pelvic infections.

Spontaneous Abortion (Miscarriage). The medical term for miscarriage is spontaneous abortion. Both of these terms mean early and unintentional termination of pregnancy before the twentieth week. After this time and before term, an early termination of pregnancy is called a stillbirth if the fetus is dead, and a premature birth if the fetus is alive. Intentional termination of pregnancy is called induced or therapeutic abortion. In conversation with patients, it is best to use the term miscarriage instead of spontaneous abortion to avoid confusion.

Spontaneous abortion occurs because the fetus has died. There are many causes of fetal death, including severe developmental abnormalities, chromosomal abnormalities, defects in the placenta, severe infection in the mother, and diabetes mellitus in the mother. Spontaneous abortion rarely occurs as a result of trauma alone. It occurs most often in the first 14 weeks of pregnancy.

There are several different forms of spontaneous abortion. A threatened abortion occurs when there is vaginal bleeding and cramping early in pregnancy, but the cervical os is closed and the fetus remains alive.

With extra caution on the part of the mother, the pregnancy often proceeds normally after a threatened miscarriage. An inevitable abortion occurs when the fetus has already died. The cervical os is open, and bleeding and cramping occur. In such cases, nothing can be done.

An incomplete spontaneous abortion is one in which some of the material from the pregnancy (the placenta, for example), remains in the uterus. In a missed spontaneous abortion, the fetus has died but there are no symptoms to indicate this.

The most common symptom of spontaneous abortion is vaginal bleeding, which may be sudden or preceded by a brown discharge, and may consist of just a few drops or a heavy flow. This sometimes occurs before a woman even knows she is pregnant, and may be mistaken for normal menstrual bleeding. In an inevitable or an incomplete spontaneous abortion, pain may accompany the bleeding. In a missed spontaneous abortion, there may be no symptoms, but the early signs of pregnancy may disappear and the uterus will not grow as it normally would in pregnancy.

Treatment for spontaneous abortion usually includes dilatation and curettage or use of a suction machine to remove any material that may be left behind in the uterus. If it is not removed, this dead tissue can cause bleeding and infection. In most cases, the only other treatment is rest. The patient often is depressed by the termination of her pregnancy, and needs emotional support.

After 6 to 8 weeks, most women who have had a spontaneous abortion can conceive again. Women who have had several consecutive spontaneous abortions may have an underlying disorder that can be found and corrected. In some cases, repeated spontaneous abortions are the result of genetic abnormalities in one or both parents.

Incompetent Cervix. This is an uncommon disorder in which the cervix does not remain closed during pregnancy. After about the fourteenth week of pregnancy, when the fetus is large enough to exert a strain on the cervix, the cervix opens and allows the contents of the uterus to fall out, thus ending the pregnancy. It is not known why this occurs.

If **incompetent cervix** is suspected, there are two procedures that can be used to strengthen the cervix early in pregnancy, called the Shirodkar-Barter technique, and the McDonald-Hofmeister technique. Both procedures involve suturing or sewing the cervix closed, so that it remains closed until term. At 38 weeks of gestation or when labor begins, the sutures may be cut to allow the cervix to open. Or, especially in the Shirodkar-Barter technique, the sutures may remain in place and the patient delivered by cesarean section.

Placenta Previa. In **placenta previa (PREE vee ah),** the placenta forms in the lower part of the uterine wall instead of in the midsection of the uterus. Sometimes the placenta actually forms over the cervix. In some cases, as the uterus grows, the placenta appears to move higher and a normal pregnancy and delivery are possible. In other cases, the placenta remains in the lower section of the uterus. This makes the placenta vulnerable to damage and to separation from the uterine wall. It also makes normal vaginal delivery difficult, since the placenta is in the way.

The main symptom of this condition is vaginal bleeding late in pregnancy. The bleeding is usually painless. If the placenta is not disturbed or damaged, there may be no symptoms at all until delivery. The problem can be identified by an ultrasound scan, which shows the location of the fetus and the placenta.

Treatment depends on the severity, whether or not the placenta has been damaged, and fetal maturity when the problem is discovered. If severe bleeding has occurred, blood transfusions may be necessary. If the cervical opening is blocked, the fetus may have to be delivered by cesarean section.

Abruptio Placentae. This situation is premature separation of the placenta from the uterine wall. It can be mild, moderate, or severe. In severe cases, the placenta is completely dislodged and the fetus almost always dies. The mother has severe pain and internal bleeding, and may quickly go into shock. In moderate cases, one-fourth to two-thirds of the placenta separates from the uterus. The uterus contracts without relaxing between contractions, and labor usually begins within 2 hours. The fetus may be affected and the mother may have both internal and external bleeding. In mild cases, slight bleeding may be the only symptom, and the fetus is not apparently affected.

In moderate to severe cases of **abruptio placentae (ab RUP shee oh pla CEN tee)**, the fetus is usually delivered as quickly as possible and blood transfusions are given to the mother as needed. The delivery may have to be by cesarean section. In mild cases, if the fetus is fully developed, labor may be induced. Otherwise, the mother is advised to rest and watch for any further bleeding until term or until any additional symptoms occur.

Pregnancy-Induced Hypertension (PIH, Toxemia, or Preeclampsia). This condition is characterized by high blood pressure, edema (fluid retention), and protein in the urine, which develop after 22 weeks of pregnancy. The cause is unknown. The condition can cause convulsions in late pregnancy. The problem can reduce the efficiency of the placenta and affect fetal growth. It can also be life-threatening for the mother, in extreme cases.

Preeclampsia may cause no symptoms at first, so blood pressure should be checked regularly. In the last weeks of pregnancy, the condition becomes increasingly severe, with swollen ankles, headaches, vomiting, blurred vision, and aversion to bright light. These symptoms can lead to eclampsia and unconsciousness (see Figure 36).

If preeclampsia is diagnosed relatively early in pregnancy and in its mildest form, treatment is usually by bed rest and possibly restriction (not elimination) of salt intake. If the condition is severe or if it occurs close to term, labor is usually induced and the fetus delivered as soon as possible. If eclampsia occurs, measures are taken to control seizures and then delivery is by the most judicious method.

Hyperemesis Gravidarum. In **hyperemesis gravidarum (HY per EM eh sis grah vih DAH rum)**, nausea and vomiting may persist past the first trimester of pregnancy, and become so severe that the pregnant woman is unable to eat or drink. Treatment for this condition usually requires hospitalization. The vomiting may be controlled by drugs. Dehydration and lack of nutrition are corrected with intravenous feedings until the patient is able to eat again. The problem may have an underlying physical or emotional cause, and the physician will attempt to discover and treat this underlying problem once the patient's nutritional balance is restored.

Maternal Diseases Affecting the Fetus
Diabetes Mellitus. Diabetes mellitus **(dy ah BEE teez meh LY tus)** is an inherited meta-

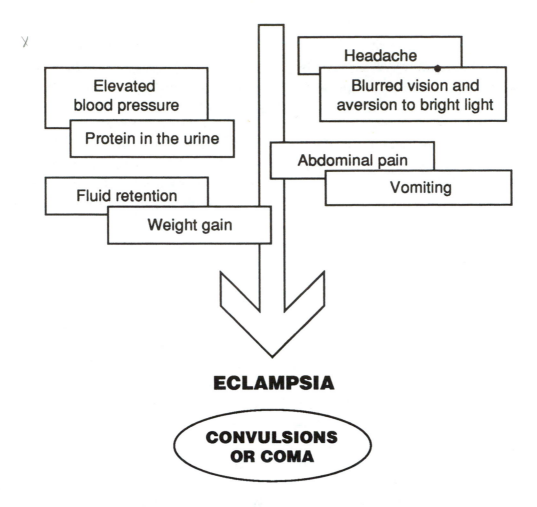

Figure 36: Symptoms of untreated pregnancy-induced hypertension.

bolic disease in which an inadequate supply of the hormone insulin is produced by the pancreas. This affects the body's ability to metabolize glucose, which in turn puts a strain on the entire body, especially the cardiovascular system. About 2 to 5 percent of pregnancies in diabetics end in the death of the fetus. Many women develop the disease for the first time during a pregnancy, so it is important that every pregnant woman be tested for diabetes.

A woman who has diabetes is usually hospitalized early in pregnancy for a complete evaluation of the status of the disease. Thereafter, every effort is made to keep the problem under control with a strict diet and sometimes injections of insulin. Toward the end of the pregnancy, a diabetic will probably be seen by the doctor more often than other patients, to be sure both mother and fetus are healthy. The chances of premature labor, abruptio placentae, and pregnancy-induced hypertension are much higher than usual for women with diabetes, so blood pressure and vaginal bleeding are carefully monitored. With severe diabetes, labor is usually induced early.

Infections. Certain infections in the mother can cross the placental barrier and cause infection in the fetus as well. At certain times in pregnancy, particularly during the first trimester, such infections can cause fetal death or severe fetal malformations, including deafness, blindness, congenital heart disorders, and mental retardation. Often the infection is very mild in the mother, as in rubella, or German measles. Other examples of diseases that can cross the placenta are toxoplasmosis, AIDS, syphilis, and cytomegalovirus.

Infections in the mother can also affect the fetus indirectly. For example, if the mother has pneumonia and is having trouble getting enough oxygen into her lungs, the fetus may also be deprived of oxygen.

Dystocia (Complications of Labor and Childbirth)

When the time comes for the child to be delivered, even a pregnancy that has been normal all along can develop problems. Abnormal labor and childbirth are called **dystocia (dis TOH see ah).**

Malpresentation. In the last weeks of pregnancy, the fetus lightens, or settles into the birth position. Normally, the fetus settles head first into the lower part of the uterus, with the face to the mother's spine. But sometimes the presenting part is the buttocks, or the fetus may be facing the wrong way. These abnormalities are called malpresentation. They can cause stress on the baby and the mother. Sometimes forceps are used to facilitate delivery and sometimes delivery by cesarean section is indicated, as in women with breech presentations (buttocks or legs first) who are having their first baby. Figure 37 illustrates different breech positions.

Abnormal Uterine Contractions. Sometimes the contractions of the uterus are either too weak or too irregular to push the baby out in the normal way. The contractions can some-times be stimulated with drugs if labor is excessively long, or delivery may have to be assisted with forceps or done by cesarean section.

Disproportion. Sometimes the baby's head is too large to pass through the mother's pelvic cavity easily. This can occur if the mother has a very small skeleton, if the baby's head is large, or possibly if the mother has had a broken pelvis at some time. In such cases, fetal monitoring devices may be attached to the baby to monitor signs of distress such as changes in heartbeat. If normal delivery appears to be impossible, or if the fetus is in trouble, delivery may have to be done by cesarean section.

Prolapsed Umbilical Cord. Occasionally, especially in cases of malpresentation, the umbilical cord precedes the fetus out of the birth canal. When this occurs, the cord can be compressed by being caught between the cervix and the fetus. This can cause fetal death if nourishment is cut off for a period of time.

To prevent prolapse, the heartbeat of the fetus is monitored constantly and every attempt is made to protect the cord. If the cord is compressed, immediate delivery by cesarean section may be necessary.

Premature Labor. Premature labor is defined as labor that occurs before the 37th week of pregnancy and/or results in an infant who weighs less than 2,500 gm. Approximately 10 to 15 percent of pregnancies in the United States end in premature labor, which is dangerous for both mother and child. Modern medicine has developed sophisticated methods of caring for premature babies, but the risks of abnormality and death remain high.

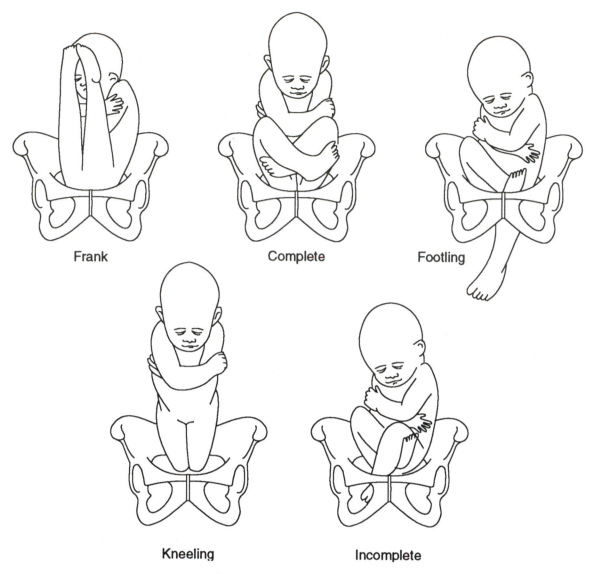

Figure 37: Five types of breech presentations.

Causes of prematurity include premature rupture of the membranes, multiple pregnancies such as twins and triplets, abnormalities in the placenta, cardiovascular and other disorders in the mother, and abnormalities in the fetus.

A common problem of premature infants is respiratory distress syndrome. The newborn is unable to breathe normally, either because the lungs are not yet fully developed or for some other reason. Emergency resuscitation is required, and the baby may have to have help from a mechanical respirator to breathe, sometimes for several weeks.

When a risk of premature delivery is detected, every effort is made to maintain the pregnancy as long as possible. Situations in which the lives of the mother and/or the fetus are in danger, such as severe preeclampsia or eclampsia, are exceptions to this rule. Bed rest is usually required and drugs may also be prescribed to delay labor. If delivery cannot be delayed, special precautions are taken. If possible, the patient is transferred to a medical center equipped with a special nursery for premature infants. If the position of the fetus is a difficult one for normal delivery, cesarean section may be necessary.

Cesarean Section. This procedure has been mentioned several times in connection with difficult or hazardous births. Cesarean section **(seh SAY ree an),** or C-section, is, in essence, the surgical removal of a fetus from the mother. This method of delivery may be necessary when normal delivery poses high risks for the mother and/or the fetus. However, the procedure is major surgery, and therefore has its own risks. Also, recovery from the operation usually takes longer than recovery from ordinary childbirth, partly because the incision takes time to heal. In most cases, normal vaginal delivery is preferred if it is possible.

At one time, it was assumed that a woman who was delivered by cesarean section could not have a normal delivery at a later date, but would have to deliver any future children in the same way. Current cesarean procedure involves a horizontal incision (called a bikini cut), does not weaken the uterus, and allows for subsequent vaginal birth.

PAIN RELIEF IN LABOR

The pain of labor varies considerably from patient to patient. It is not clear exactly what causes the pain physiologically, but it is associated with uterine muscle contractions. The patient's previous experience, experiences related by her mother and her friends, her level of anxiety about the birth, and her understanding of the process of labor and childbirth all affect her individual response.

Anesthetics, which cause lack of feeling, and analgesics, which reduce sensitivity to pain, can be given during labor but must be used cautiously. Heavy use of either type of drug can prolong labor and endanger the fetus. Successful labor usually requires a conscious effort by the mother to push down along with the contractions, in the second stage of labor. A heavily sedated patient cannot perform this function effectively. Some drugs also can cause depression of the mother's breathing, which reduces the oxygen the fetus is receiving. Finally, some drugs cross the placenta and directly affect fetal function. For these reasons, the patient should be awake and alert during delivery and administration of pain medications must be carefully timed and chosen and exactly placed.

A pudendal **(pyoo DEN dal)** block may be given to provide local pain relief in the vaginal area. This is often done before the use of forceps to aid delivery, or before an episiotomy, or incision to widen the vaginal opening. Another technique that may be used in the first stage of labor is epidural **(EP ih dur al)** anesthesia. In this procedure, a painkiller is injected into the spinal column to deaden sensation in the lower part of the body.

Many women have found that by using breathing and relaxation techniques, changing positions, having the support of a labor partner, and using other techniques taught at prepared-childbirth classes, they can greatly reduce or eliminate the need for anesthetic intervention.

Fill in the blanks.

1. The normal gestation time for full development of a human being is _____ .

2. Both methods of estimating the due date assume that ovulation occurred

   _____ .

3. Even before the first missed period blood or urine can be tested for _____ , which is secreted by the placenta.

4. The exchange of oxygen, nutrients, and waste materials occurs through the

   _____ membrane.

5. The fluid in which the developing embryo or fetus floats until just before birth is called

   _____ fluid.

6. The placenta is made up of connective tissue and endothelial tissue that support a network of _____ .

7. The _____ secretes HCG, which stimulates the corpus luteum, which produces progesterone and estrogen to maintain the uterine lining.

8. Between the eighth and eleventh weeks of development the embryo becomes a

   _____ .

9. The time during which the organs are developing is the time the embryo is most susceptible to _____ .

10. The stage of development mentioned in Question 9 is called the _____ of pregnancy.

11. Three methods of monitoring fetal growth and development are:

    a. _____

    b. _____

    c. _____

12. An expectant mother's back pain may be associated with the fact that the ligaments that hold the joints to the skeleton become more _____ .

13. Unlike Braxton-Hicks contractions, which are irregular and uncoordinated, labor contractions are _____ and _____ .

14. The _____ is expelled from the uterus during the third stage of labor.

15. The uterus also contracts to prevent _____ .

16. The two hormones involved in lactation are _____ from the posterior pituitary and _____ from the anterior pituitary.

17. The Apgar score assesses five signs. What are they?

    a. _____

    b. _____

(continued next page)

c. _____

d. _____

e. _____

18. The score is recorded at _____ and _____ minutes after birth.

19. In general, pregnant women are told to avoid _____ , _____ , and _____ to reduce the possibilities of congenital defects.

20. When the fertilized egg implants outside the uterus, the pregnancy is called

    _____ .

21. Unintentional termination of a pregnancy before the twentieth week is called

    _____ or_____ .

22. The premature separation of the placenta from the uterine wall is known as

    _____ .

23. Three examples of diseases that cross the placenta are:

    a. _____

    b. _____

    c. _____

24. A common problem of premature infants is _____ , because their lungs have not yet fully developed.

Short answers.

25. What is Chadwick's sign? _____

26. What is a zygote? _____

27. Why is the mother's intake of protein especially important in the third trimester?

    _____

28. A premature infant is defined as _____ .

29. Parturition may be defined as _____ .

30. Cervical effacement is _____ .

31. Three factors that increase the risk of ectopic pregnancies are _____

    _____ .

32. How might an umbilical cord become prolapsed? _____

    _____

33. What are three of the dangers associated with the use of anesthetics during labor?

    a. _____

    b. _____

    c. _____

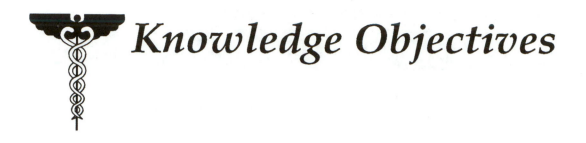

Knowledge Objectives

After completing this chapter, you should be able to:

- define the terms contraception, abortion, and sterilization
- list two different natural birth control methods and describe their advantages and disadvantages
- list six artificial birth control methods and describe their advantages and disadvantages
- describe techniques that may be used to cause abortion
- describe two methods of female sterilization

Contraception and Sterilization

INTRODUCTION

Contraception (KON trah SEP shun) can be defined as temporary prevention of pregnancy. **Sterilization (STER ih lih ZAY shun)** is permanent pregnancy prevention. Contraception deals with the opposite problem of infertility treatment. It involves ways to prevent pregnancy in a fertile woman with a fertile sex partner. There are several available methods of temporary birth control, or family planning. Each one has advantages and disadvantages that a couple must consider when choosing which method to use (see Figure 38).

NATURAL CONTRACEPTIVE METHODS

These methods do not require medications or devices that interfere with the natural process of conception. They are generally less effective than artificial methods, but some couples prefer them because of religious beliefs or for other personal reasons.

Withdrawal

In withdrawal, or **coitus interruptus (KOH ih tus in teh RUP tus)**, the man withdraws his penis from the woman's vagina during intercourse, before ejaculation. This theoretically prevents sperm from entering the woman's body and fertilizing an ovum. It requires excellent control and timing on the part of the man, and it may decrease sexual satisfaction for one or both partners. Also, it is possible for sperm to enter the vagina either before ejaculation or from semen ejaculated near the vaginal opening.

This method of birth control involves no cost and has no medical side effects. It is considered 75 to 80 percent effective.

Rhythm Method

The **rhythm method** is based on avoidance of intercourse during times when the woman is most likely to be fertile. The woman keeps records of her monthly cycle and calculates the days when she will probably ovulate. If the ovum can be fertilized for only 24 hours after it is released from the ovary, if sperm live for only 48 hours after ejaculation, and if the woman's menstrual cycle is regular, it is theoretically possible to prevent conception by avoiding intercourse during the "unsafe" time of the month.

Unfortunately, every woman has irregu-

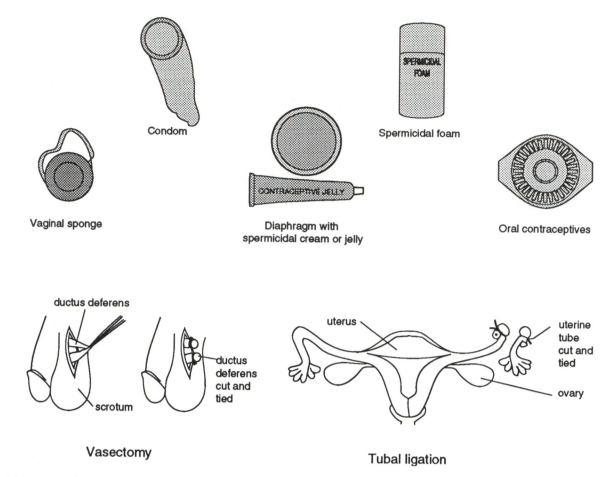

Figure 38: Current contraception techniques.

lar cycles from time to time. This is why the rhythm method often fails. Also, it is possible (though unusual) for sperm to live as long as 6 days in the woman's body.

A woman can determine when she ovulates with some accuracy if she takes her temperature every morning and records it. Body temperature increases by half a degree or more at ovulation and remains high for several days. However, the "unsafe" time begins before ovulation. The couple must still estimate when ovulation will occur, and avoid intercourse before that, to avoid pregnancy.

Like withdrawal, the rhythm method is inexpensive and without medical side effects. Its disadvantages are unreliability and the necessity to carefully time all sexual act

ivity. For some couples, using rhythm means being able to have sex only a few days out of a month. The effectiveness of the rhythm method of birth control is rated at 60 to 85 percent.

ARTIFICIAL CONTRACEPTIVE METHODS

Artificial methods of birth control include barrier devices, spermicides **(SPER mih sydz),** and oral contraceptives ("the pill"), intrauterine devices, and implants. Barriers include the condom and diaphragm, and the cervical cap. Spermicides are found in several forms, such as creams, jellies, suppositories, and foams. "The pill" contains combinations of estrogen and progesterone, hormones that affect the menstrual cycle.

Barrier Devices

Condom. The **condom** or sheath is put on the man's penis after he has an erection and before he enters the woman (see Figure 38). It is a sleeve made of thin rubber or a similar material, which fits over the penis and prevents semen from entering the woman's vagina at ejaculation. Condoms are available without a doctor's prescription. They are relatively inexpensive, have an effectiveness rate of 75 to 80 percent, and help to prevent transmission of venereal disease. One disadvantage of the condom is that it may reduce sexual pleasure for one or both partners.

Diaphragm. A **diaphragm (DY ah fram)** is a device shaped like a ring with a rubber dome over the top (see Figure 38). It is designed to fit inside the woman's vagina, over the cervix. Diaphragms prevent sperm from entering the cervical canal and uterus. A diaphragm must be fitted to the individual patient by a physician. If it is the wrong size, it will not prevent pregnancy and it may also be uncomfortable. The diaphragm should be used with a spermicidal cream or jelly. It is inserted into the vagina before intercourse and should be left in place for at least 8 hours afterward. A new application of spermicide should be made before each act of intercourse.

Diaphragm users should examine them periodically by running water into them. Even a pinhole can make the diaphragm ineffective. Also, the user should know how to apply spermicide to the diaphragm, how to insert it properly, and how to check its position. When used correctly, the diaphragm and spermicide combination is 75 to 85 percent effective in preventing pregnancy.

The cervical cap is similar to the diaphragm, except that it is smaller and is placed directly over the cervix.

Spermicides

Spermicides are sometimes used in combination with either a condom or a diaphragm, but they can be used alone (see Figure 38). Some condoms come precoated with a spermicidal agent. Creams, jellies, foam, and suppositories of spermicide are available, without prescription. Used alone they are about 75 percent effective in killing sperm and thus preventing pregnancy. When used in combination with a barrier method, they can be up to 85 percent effective. In some cases, these preparations can cause irritation of the tender skin of either partner, or even allergic reactions. Also, these agents tend to be messy, and they must be reapplied for each act of intercourse.

Intrauterine Devices (IUDs).

An **intrauterine device**, or IUD, is a flexible piece of wire or plastic that is inserted into the woman's uterus. IUDs somehow prevent any fertilized ovum from implanting itself in the uterine wall.

While the IUD enjoyed a high degree of contraceptive success, manufacturers have removed most IUDs from the market after being bombarded with problems including uterine perforation and pelvic inflammatory disease which can both lead to sterility if improperly diagnosed and treated.

Oral Contraceptives

Oral contraceptives are the most effective method of birth control, but they also have the greatest potential for side effects (see Figure 38). However, low-dose pills have reduced the risk of blood clots and cardiovascular disorders. The pill may protect against ovarian or endometrial cancer. It also generally reduces menstrual flow and menstrual cramps (dysmenorrhea).

The pill is composed of different combinations and dosages of the sex hormones estrogen and progesterone. By increasing the amounts of these substances in the body at certain points in the cycle, the pill prevents follicle development and ovulation. It also inhibits the release of FSH and LH by the pituitary gland. Since there is no ovum available to be fertilized, intercourse does not result in pregnancy. The pill has proved to be 99 percent effective.

To achieve this level of effectiveness, the patient must take the pills exactly according to instructions. Some types are taken daily, some are taken for 21 days, then discontinued for 7 days to allow for the monthly shedding of the uterine lining. Some oral contraceptives include 21 hormone pills and seven placebos, or pills with no medication in them. Some women find it easier to follow the medication schedule if they can take a pill each day without interruption. If a patient forgets to take one or more pills in a cycle, she may not be protected in that month and she should use an additional contraceptive method to be sure.

Contraceptive Implant

A recently approved method of contraception is the contraceptive implant (Norplant). The implant consists of six steroid-containing capsules. The implant prevents ovulation by releasing progestin and levonorgestrel slowly into the bloodstream.

The capsules are inserted under the skin, under local anesthesia. Insertion requires 5 to 10 minutes and contraceptive effects begin 24 hours after implantation. The implants are effective for 5 years. They must be removed when contraception is no longer required or replaced at the end of 5 years.

The major side effect is irregular bleeding (spotting). Other side effects include slight weight gain and rare infections of the insertion site. The Norplant implant has a high rate of effectiveness that surpasses that of the pill or the IUD.

ABORTION

As a method of birth control, **abortion** is controversial. Some people consider abortion to be the moral equivalent of murder. Others consider it a legitimate and sometimes necessary means of family planning. Therapeutic abortion or induced abortion may be done to preserve the life or health of the pregnant woman, when a medical condition makes pregnancy dangerous for her.

Pregnancies are sometimes terminated in this way when amniocentesis establishes that a fetus is abnormal, as in Down's syndrome and other genetic disorders. Abortions are usually done during the first trimester (first 3 months) of pregnancy. Early in pregnancy, an abortion can usually be performed by aspiration. In this procedure, the contents of the uterus are removed with a suction device. A pregnancy can also be terminated by a D&C (dilatation and curettage) procedure. Later in pregnancy, abortions can be done by dilatation and evacuation (D&E), which is similar to a D&C but more complicated. It is also possible to perform an abortion by inducing labor, or initiating labor by artificial means. This is done only if it is too late in the pregnancy to use one of the other methods. It is rarely done because of the risks to the mother and the possibility that the fetus may be viable, or able to survive outside the womb.

Although techniques and equipment for abortion have been refined considerably in recent years, and abortions can be performed legally under various circumstances in different states by trained personnel instead of illegally, there are still risks of complications. These include abnormal bleeding, perforation of the uterus, and other damage to the reproductive system that may prevent later pregnancies. There is also a risk of infection if material from the fetus or placenta is left in the uterus.

STERILIZATION

There are two general methods of female sterilization: **tubal ligation (ly GAY shun)**, in which the uterine tubes are severed, and hysterectomy, in which the uterus is removed. Hysterectomy is not usually done for this reason alone, but a physician may recommend it for a woman who has other reproductive-tract problems and does not want to have children.

Tubal ligation can be done in several ways: immediately after delivery, or as a separate procedure. As a separate procedure it is done in an outpatient setting and does not require an overnight stay. Laparoscopic tubal ligation is done by a small incision in the navel through which a scope is passed and through which the tubes are cut, tied, and often burned or cauterized.

Male sterilization is a much less complicated procedure called a **vasectomy (vah SECK toh mee)**. It usually requires about 20 minutes to cut or cauterize the vas deferens and is done in a medical office.

These sterilization methods are totally effective, which is why more than one-third of couples use one of them. Once the procedure is complete, it usually cannot be reversed even though new microsurgery techniques have made repair of the tubes possible in a few cases, but the operation is expensive with a success rate of 15 percent.

STOP AND REVIEW

Fill in the blanks.

1. The diaphragm and cervical cap both fit over the _____ .

2. Oral contraceptives inhibit the release of _____ and _____ from the pituitary gland.

3. A pregnancy can be terminated by a D&C, which means _____ and _____ .

4. Two methods of female sterilization are:

   a. _____

   b. _____

Short answers.

5. How can a woman determine when she ovulates? _____

6. How does the IUD prevent pregnancy? _____

7. How do oral contraceptives prevent pregnancy? _____

8. _____ is a sterilization procedure in which the uterine tubes are cut, tied, and sometimes burned.

9. Male sterilization is called a _____ .

Abortion Intentional termination of pregnancy.

Abruptio placentae Premature detachment of a placenta.

Acid-base balance Maintenance of the pH of the blood at 7.35 to 7.45 (slightly alkaline).

Acrosome Cap on the head of the sperm; it is specially formed to penetrate an ovum.

Active transport Transport of substances between cells by means of the energy released by chemical reactions in a cell.

Acute kidney failure See Intrarenal failure, postrenal failure, prerenal failure, vascular renal failure.

Acute pyelonephritis Infection of the tissue surrounding the nephons, usually caused by a bladder infection moving up the ureters to the kidney.

Adrenal gland Endocrine gland located on top of the kidney.

Afferent arteriole Branch of an interlobular artery that carried blood to the renal corpuscles.

AIDS (Acquired Immune Deficiency Syndrome) Disease that starts by a virus which affects the body's immune system.

Aldosterone Hormone secreted by the adrenal glands that increases the amount of sodium reabsorbed by the distal tubules, and thus the amount of water moving through the tubule walls by osmosis. Sodium and thus water are conserved.

Amenorrhea Absence of menstruation.

Amniocentesis Test that evaluates fetal well-being by examining a sample of amniotic fluid.

Amnion Inner layer of the placenta.

Antidiuretic hormone (ADH) Hormone secreted by the pituitary gland, that circulates in the blood, causing distal and collecting tubules to become permeable to water, thus increasing reabsorption of water and decreasing urination.

Anuria Complete lack of urine excretion.

Apgar scoring system System for rapidly evaluating a newborn's health at 1 and 5 minutes after birth.

Areola Circular area of a different color surrounding the nipple.

Aspiration Procedure in which fluid is removed with a needle, for testing or to relieve pressure.

B

Balanitis Irritation or infection of the foreskin and/or the outer surface of the glans penis.

Balanitis xerotica obliterans Condition in which the tip of the penis dries and shrivels, causing stricture of the urethral meatus.

Benign enlargement of the prostate Part of the aging process, in which extra deposits of normal prostate tissue enlarge the gland.

Benign prostatic hypertrophy See Benign enlargement of the prostate.

Bilateral salpingo-oophorectomy Surgical removal of the uterine tubes and ovaries, which often accompanies hysterectomy.

Biophysical profile Test to evaluate fetal well-being based on fetal breathing, gross body movement, and muscle tone as well as amniotic fluid volume.

Bladder A membranous sac. Also, organ that stores urine until it is excreted from the body.

Bladder stone A vesical calculus. Stone similar to kidney stones, that forms in the bladder.

Blastocyst Hollow, fluid-filled balls of cells formed from the morula.

Bowman's capsule Doubled-walled tubular cup at the beginning of the nephron that contains the glomerulus.

Braxton-Hicks contractions Irregular uterine muscle contractions that prepare the body for labor and delivery.

Bulbourethral gland or Cowper's glands One of a pair of pea-sized glands below the prostate; they secrete a mucoid part of the semen.

C

Calyx (calyces) A cup-shaped organ or cavity. In the kidney, a duct connecting a medullary pyramid with the renal pelvis.

Candidiasis Vaginal infection with candida yeast.

Cast Tiny cylindrical bit of material formed in the kidney tubules of protein and other material.

Catheter A tubular instrument for withdrawing fluids from a cavity; also, one of a number of instruments used to diagnose and treat urinary problems.

Cavernous portion of the urethra Part of the urethra that passes through cavernous (erectile dilatable spaces which fill with blood) tissue.

Cells of Leydig Specialized cells in the testes that make the male sex hormone testosterone.

Cervical dysplasia Development of abnormal cells on the cervix, an early sign of cancer.

Cervical erosion Growth of columnar epithelial tissue over the cervix.

Cervical polyps Common tumor of the cervix, composed of mucus-producing tissue.

Cervix Lower and narrow end of the uterus.

Chancroid Sexually transmitted infection that produces lesions on the genitals.

Chlamydia Microscopic parasites which can cause NSU.

Chordee Abnormal downward curvature of the penis.

Chorion Outer layer of the placenta.

Chorionic vili Threadlike projections from the chorion.

Chronic kidney failure Gradual loss of kidney function over a period of time, caused by repeated infections or by other chronic diseases.

Chronic pyelonephritis Inflammation of the tissue surrounding the nephrons, caused by repeated, undetected urinary tract infections, arising from such problems as reflux or kidney or bladder stones.

Cilia Hairlike projections, as on the inner wall of the uterine tube.

Circumcision Surgical removal of all or part of the foreskin.

Clitoris Small erectile body that is part of the external female genitalia.

Coitus interruptus Contraceptive method in which the man withdraws his penis before ejaculation.

Colostrum Thin, yellow milky fluid secreted from the breasts a few days after delivery.

Colporrhaphy Surgical tightening of weakened pelvic muscles.

Colposcope Instrument inserted into the vagina to magnify and examine the cervix.

Condom Sheath that fits over an erect penis and is used to prevent pregnancy.

Conization Removal of a cone-shaped tissue sample from the cervix.

Contraception Temporary prevention of pregnancy.

Contraceptive implant Steriod-containing capsules that are implanted under the woman's skin to prevent pregnancy.

Cowper's gland See Bulbourethral gland.

Cortex (of the kidney) Outer portion of the kidney.

Creatinine clearance test Spectrophotometer test of a 24-hour urine specimen, to discover how much creatinine was excrete during that period. A test of kidney efficiency.

Cryptorchidism Undescended testes.

Cystitis Urinary bladder inflammation.

Cystocele Bladder protrusion into the vagina.

Cystography X-ray procedure in which an opaque solution is injected into the bladder, and pictures are taken.

Cystoscope Tube with a light source and lens system in its end, designed for viewing the inside of the urethra and bladder.

D

Detrusor muscle Muscle that opens the internal sphincter in the bladder.

Diaphragm Barrier contraceptive that fits over the cervix.

Diffusion Movement of molecules from a higher to a lower concentration, usually through a semipermeable membrane.

Dysmenorrhea Painful menstrual periods; menstrual cramps.

Dystocia Abnormal labor and childbirth.

Dysuria Painful or difficult urination.

E

Ectopic pregnancy Pregnancy in which the fertilized egg is implanted outside the uterus.

Edema Swelling due to fluid accumulation in the tissues.

Effacement Softening and thinning of the cervix in preparation for labor and delivery.

Efferent arteriole Narrower branch of an arteriole leaving the glomerulus, functions to increase blood pressure in the glomerulus.

Ejaculation A sudden act of explusion. Automatic muscle contractions along the length of the urethra that push semen out of the penis.

Ejaculatory duct One of a pair of ducts leading from the junction of the seminal vesicles and the vas deferens to the top of the urethra.

Electrolyte Chemical compound that ionizes charged particles in solution.

Electrolyte balance Regulation of levels of electrolytes such as sodium, potassium, and calcium in the bloodstream.

Emission A discharge, specifically reflex movement of semen into the urethra.

Embryo Developing fertilized ovum from weeks two through eight of gestation.

Endometriosis Disorder in which endometrial tissue grows in locations other than the inner lining of the uterus.

Endometrium Inner wall of the uterus.

End-stage kidney disease Final stage of kidney failure, when chronic kidney failure becomes so severe that the kidneys cannot keep the patient functioning.

Epididymis One of a pair of structures containing a coiled tubule about 6 m long; it is attached to the side of the testis and serves as a collection and storage place for sperm; it leads into the vas deferens.

Epididymitis Inflammation and swelling of the epididymis.

Episiotomy Surgical cut in the perineum during childbirth to prevent irregular tears and make delivery easier.

Epispadias Congenital abnormality of the penis, including misplacement of the urinary meatus and chordee. The urethra opens on the dorsum of the penis.

Erectile tissue Tissue in the penis, full of arteries and veins that can engorge with blood upon sexual stimulation, causing an erection.

Erection The condition of being made rigid and elevated. Enlargement and stiffening of the penis, due to engorgement of the erectile tissue with blood.

Escherichia coli Normal intestinal bacteria that can cause lower urinary tract infections.

Estrogen Hormone produced in the ovaries, adrenal cortex, testes, and fetoplacental unit.

External sphincter Muscle surrounding the opening fro the urethra to the outside.

External urinary meatus Urethral opening at the tip of the glans penis.

Extracellular fluid See Interstitial fluid.

F

FSH See Follicle-stimulating hormone.

Fallopian tube See Uterine tube.

Fetus Developing human from about the ninth week of gestation to birth.

Fibroadenoma Common benign breast tumor.

Fibrocystic disease Common benign breast disease that causes breast lumps and tenderness and sometimes nipple discharge.

Fibroids Benign tumors of the uterus.

Filtrate A liquid which has passed through a filter. Fluid filtered out of the blood into Bowman's capsule, that is made up of water, solutes, and waste products.

Fimbriae Finger-like projections of the uterine tube that sweep across the ovary and move the ovum into the tube.

Flagellum In sperm, the tail that provides motility.

Flank pain Severe pain in the sides above the ilium and below the ribs.

Fluid balance Equilibrium between intake and excretion of fluids in the body.

Follicle-stimulating hormone (FSH) Gonadotropin produced by the pituitary that stimulate sperm production in males and estrogen secretion in females.

Follicular phase Phase of menstrual cycle during which hormones stimulate the ovarian follicles to actively secrete estrogen.

Foreskin Loose fold of skin over the glans penis.

Fundus Top part of uterus.

G

Gestation Period of time from ovum fertilization to birth.

Glans penis Expansion of corpus spongiosum at the tip of the penis, containing the external urinary meatus (urethral opening).

Glomerular filtration Part of the process of urine formation in which blood from the renal artery flows into the glomerulus and the fluid is filtered out into Bowman's capsule; it involves active transport of sodium into the peritubular capillaries and movement of water in the kidney tubules (by osmosis) into the blood.

Glomerulonephritis Infection of the nephrons (especially the glomeruli) of the kidneys characterized by inflammation of capillaries.

Glomerulus Network of capillaries within a nephron.

Gonorrhea Sexually transmitted contagious inflammation of the genital mucous membrane that can affect the urinary tract, caused by neisseria gonorrhoeae.

Graafian follicle Ripe ovarian follicle.

H

Head In sperm, the end full of genetic material and nitochondria.

Hematuria Blood in the urine.

Hemospermia Blood in the semen.

Hilus A depression at that part of an organ where the vessels and nerves enter; center of the concave area of the kidney.

HIV Human autoimmunne deficiency virus which infects the cells that protect the body against invasion of pathogens.

Hyrdocele Accumulation of abnormal amounts of lubricating fluid around the testicle or along the spermatic cord.

Hydrocelectomy Surgical removal of hydrocele.

Hydronephrosis Excess fluid in the kidney.

Hymen Membrane that partially covers the vaginal opening in a young woman who has not had sexual intercourse.

Hyperemesis gravidarum Persistent vomiting during pregnancy.

Hyperkalemia Excess potassium in the blood that can be caused by kidney failure, tissue damage, or acidosis.

Hypernatremia Excess sodium in the blood that can be caused by insufficient fluid intake, ADH deficiency, and excess adrenocortical hormones.

Hypernephroma Invasive kidney tumor.

Hypokalemia Insufficient potassium in the blood, caused by dietary deficiency, dehydration, alkalosis, or certain diuretic drugs.

Hyponatremia Insufficient sodium in the blood, caused by trauma, surgery, cirrhosis, and other disorders.

Hypospadias Congenital abnormality of the penis in which the urethra opens on the underside of the penis and also includes chordee, misplacement of the urinary meatus, abnormal smallness, and sometimes the presence of a partial or complete vagina and uterus.

Hysterectomy Surgical removal of the uterus.

Hysterosalpingography X-ray study in which radiopaque dye in the female reproductive system reveals obstructions and other abnormalities.

I

ICSH See Interstitial cell-stimulating hormone.

Impotence Inability either to achieve or to maintain an erection.

Incompetent cervix Inability of the cervix to remain closed during pregnancy.

Incontinence Involuntary release of urine, which may be acute (transient) or persistent (established).

Indwelling catheter Catheter implanted in a patient for a peiod of time, to replace the normal passageway for urine.

Infertility Inability to produce offspring.

Inguinal canal One of two openings in the lower abdominal wall through which the vas deferens passes.

Interlobular artery Branch of the renal artery situated between lobules.

Interlobular vein Vein carrying blood away from the nephron and to the renal vein situated between lobules.

Internal sphincter In the bladder, the circular smooth muscle surrounding the opening from the bladder to the urethra.

Interstitial fluid Fluid appearing between the cells.

Interstitial cell-stimulating hormone (ICSH) Gonadotropin produced by the pituitary that stimulates production of testosterone by stimulating the cells of Leydig.

Intracellular fluid Fluid inside a cell.

Intrarenal failure Kidney failure caused by damage to the kidney itself, from infection or other causes.

Intrauterine device (IUD) Flexible wire or plastic device that is inserted into the uterus to prevent pregnancy.

Intravenous pyelogram X-ray procedure, used to visualize the kidney. The progress of a dye, that has been injected into the patient's vein, through the kidneys is photographed in a series of pictures over several hours.

Involution Process by which the uterus returns to its usual size and shape after pregnancy.

J

"Jock itch" Rash and severe itching of the genitals caused by such things as fungal infections and allergic reactions.

K

Kidney cyst Fluid-filled sac that appears in the kidney.

Kidney dialysis Artificial replacement of kidney function, either outside the body with an artificial kidney (hemodialysis) or inside the body (peritoneal dialysis) by means of a solution called dialysate which uses the peritoneal membrane for the exchange of fluids and electrolytes.

Kidney failure See Chronic kidney failure, intrarenal failure, postrenal failure, prerenal failure, vascular renal failure.

Kidney stone Stone, usually containing calcium, that forms in the kidney calyx and usually remains on the renal pelvis. If it moves into the ureter, it can cause pain and obstruction.

Kidney transplantation Replacement of a diseased organ with one taken from an accident victim or someone who died of disorders unrelated to kidney problems, or from a relative.

L

Labia Lips of the external female genitalia; divided into labia majora (outer lips) and labia minora (inner lips).

Lactation Breast milk secretion.

Lactiferous duct Main duct that transports breast milk from the alveoli to the nipple.

Laparoscopy Examination of the interior of the abdomen via a laparoscope.

Lightening Settling of the fetus into the pelvic area 2 to 4 weeks before labor.

Lochia Uterine discharge after childbirth, which occurs in three stages.

Loop of nephron (Henle) Part of the system of tubes in the nephron in medullary portion that controls the concentration and chemical makeup of the urine.

Lower urinary tract infection Infection affecting the bladder or urethra.

Luteal phase Phase of menstrual cycle during which the ruptured follicle becomes the corpus luteum and begins to secrete progesterone.

Luteinizing hormone (LH) Hormone released from the anterior pituitary gland that stimulates ovarian follicle development in females and interstitial cell development in males.

Lymphogranuloma venereum Sexually transmitted chlamydia infection. It may lead to nondestructive elephantiasis of labia and clitoris, or of penis and scrotum, and to development of rectal stenosis or strictures.

M

Mammary duct ectasia Hardening and enlargement of mammary ducts.

Mammary glands Glandular tissue in the breasts that secrete milk.

Mammography Radiographic examination of the breast.

Mastectomy Surgical removal of the breast.

Mastitis Inflammation of the mammary gland, or breast.

Medulla Inner portion of any organ, such as the kidney or ovary.

Membranous portion of urethra Middle part of the male urethra.

Menarche First menstrual period in puberty.

Menopause Cessation of menses.

Menstrual cycle Female reproductive cycle, which typically lasts 28 days.

Menstrual phase Phase of menstrual cycle when endometrium is shed.

Micturition Voiding of urine.

Middle piece In sperm, the section just behind the head, that contains the nucleus of the sperm and mitochondria as well.

Mitosis Method of cell division in which all daughter cells have the same genetic composition as the parent cell.

Mons pubis Pad of fatty tissue above the vulva and over the pubic bone, which is covered with pubic hair.

Morula Solid ball of cells formed by mitosis of the zygote.

Myoma See Fibroids.

Myomectomy Surgical removal of fibroids.

Myometrium Muscular wall that surrounds that endometrium of the uterus.

N

NSU See Nonspecific urethritis.

Nagele's rule Method of estimating the date of delivery by counting back 3 months from the first day of the last menstrual period and then adding 7 days.

Negative feedback Process in which production of one substance (such as testosterone) reduces production of another substance (such as FSH and ICSH), and thus also the first substance; when the level of the first substance drops, the second substance is produced in greater volume and the process repeats itself.

Nephron Microscopic functioning unit of the kidney.

Nocturia Excessive urination at night.

Nonspecific urethritis (NSU) Sexually transmitted infection affecting the urethra, caused most commonly by chlamydia.

O

Oligomenorrhea Infrequent menstrual periods.

Oliguria Insufficient urine excretion.

Oogenesis Formation of ova in the ovaries.

Oogonium (oogonia) Egg germ cell.

Oral contraceptives Pills that contain estrogen and progesterone and are taken to prevent pregnancy.

Orchiectomy Surgical removal of one or both testes.

Orchiopexy Surgical procedure to move an undescended testis into the proper position.

Orchitis Inflammation of the testes.

Orgasm Ejaculation, in the male, and involuntary contraction of the perineal muscles, in the female, at the climax of sexual intercourse. Other sensory and motor responses occur simultaneously (such as increase in heartbeat).

Osmolality Level of solute concentration.

Osmosis Diffusion of a solvent (usually water) from a greater solvent concentration to lesser solvent concentration or from lesser solute concentration to greater salute concentration through a selectively permeable membrane.

Ovary One of two organs in which ova are formed in the female.

Ovulation Cyclic release of a mature ovum.

Ovum (ova) Female reproductive cell; egg.

Oxytocin Hormone that stimulates labor contractions and breast milk ejection.

P

Palliation Relief of symptoms rather than treatment of their cause.

Papanicolaou (Pap) smear Screening test for cervical cancer.

Papilla (of the kidney) A nipple-shaped projection; tip of the medullary pyramid.

Parathormone Hormone secreted by the parathyroid gland which regulates levels of calcium in the blood and urine.

Parathyroid hormone See Parathormone.

Paraurethral glands Glands that have ducts which open on either side of the urethra in women.

Parturition Act of giving birth; or labor and delivery.

Passive transport Random activity of molecules (including diffusion and osmosis) that moves fluids and solutes down their concentration gradients through a membrane without energy expenditure.

Pelvic inflammatory disease (PID) Pelvic infection that affects the vagina, uterus, uterine tubes, ovaries, and the surrounding tissues.

Penile wart Wart on the penis.

Penis Male sex organ that contains the urethra and introduces semen into the vagina.

Peristalsis Automatic successive muscle contractions that move substances through a hollow organ, as urine through the ureter.

Peritonitis Infection of the abdominal cavity.

Peritoneum Membranous sac that lines the abdominal cavity and covers the viscera.

Peritubular capillary Part of the network of capillaries surrounding the nephron.

Pessary Device inserted into the vagina to support the uterus and correct displacement.

Peyronie's disease Disease of aging in which the tissue covering the corpora cavernosa of the penis becomes fibrous, hardens, or even ossifies.

Phimosis Tightening of the foreskin in a uncircumsized male, also an analogous condition in the clitoris.

Placenta Organ that surrounds the fetus and connects it to the mother.

Placenta previa Formation of the placenta in the lower part of the uterus rather than the middle part.

Polyuria Excess urine excretion.

Postrenal failure Kidney failure caused by blockage in the ureters or in the kidney pelvis.

Poststreptococcal glomerulonephritis Infection of the nephrons (glomeruli) occurring as a complication of streptococcal infection.

Pregnancy Condition of having a developing embryo or fetus in the body as a result of the union of a sperm and an ovum.

Pregnancy-induced hypertension Condition caused by pregnancy in which the woman develops high blood pressure, edema, and protein in the urine.

Premature labor Labor that occurs before the thirty-seventh week of pregnancy or results in an infant who weights less than 2,500 gm.

Premenstrual syndrome (PMS) Cluster of symptoms, such as irritability and fluid retention, that occur before the onset of menses.

Prepuce See Foreskin.

Prerenal failure Kidney failure caused by dehydration, collapse of blood vessels to the kidney, or reduced heart output.

Priapism Unrelaxing erection that persists in the absence of a stimulus.

Progesterone Female hormone that helps prepare the uterus to receive a fertilized egg.

Prolactin Hormone that stimulates and sustains lactation.

Prostate gland Muscular gland located below the bladder and surrounding the superior portion of the male urethra; it secretes a part of the semen.

Prostatic portion of the urethra Part of the male urethra closest to the prostate gland.

Prostatitis Infection of the prostate gland.

Proximal tubule System of tubes closest to the renal corpuscle in the nephron that controls the concentration and chemical makeup of the urine.

Pyelonephritis Infection of the tissue that surrounds the nephrons.

Pyramid (medullary) A triangular structurfe in the medulla composed of the straight segments of the renal tubules.

Pyuria Presence of pus in urine.

R

Rectocele Protrusion of the rectum into the vagina.

Reflux A backward or return flow. Backflow of urine into the ureters from the bladder.

Renal artery Artery supplying blood to the kidney.

Renal calculus See Kidney stone.

Renal colic Severe, stabbing abdominal pain caused by a kidney stone passing along the ureter.

Renal column Pillar-like sections of the cortex tissue which dip into the kidney medulla.

Renal corpuscle Glomerulus and Bowman's capsule together.

Renal pelvis Expansion in the kidney at the upper end of the ureter into which the calyces open and urine is temporarily collected.

Renal threshold That concentration of a substance that is necessary in the blood before more than a normal quantity of it is eliminated in the urine.

Renal vein Vein carrying blood from the kidney.

Renin Enzyme secreted by the kidneys that triggers production of aldosterone by the adrenal glands.

Resectoscope Tubular instrument containing a light and lens system, and a cutting attachment; it is used to examine and sometimes cut away part of the prostate gland by passing through the urethra.

Retroversion Tipping backward of the uterus.

Rhythm method Contraceptive method based on avoidance of intercourse during the woman's fertile period.

Rugae In the bladder, folds of the mucous-membrane lining that allow it to stretch to accommodate urine.

S

Salpingitis Inflammation of the uterine tubes.

Scrotum Sac of loose skin suspended below the body, which contains the testes.

Semen Fluid in which sperm are carried; also contains secretion from the testes and the seminal vesicles, and alkaline fluids from the prostate and the bulbourethral glands.

Seminal vesicle One of a pair of pouch-like structures posterior and inferior to the bladder that secretes part of the semen into the ejaculatory ducts.

Seminiferous tubule Convoluted tubule in a lobe of a testis, where sperm are made by meiosis.

Solution Combination of a fluid (solvent) with substances (solutes) that are dissolved in it.

Sound Metal rod, curved at one end and with a handle at the other, used to treat stricture of the urethra.

Speculum Instrument used in a pelvic examination to widen the vagina.

Sperm Male sex cell or spermatozoon.

Spermatic cord A supporting structure extending from a testis to the inguinal ring that inclues the vas deferens, arteries, veins, lymphatics, nerves, cremaster muscle, and connective tissue.

Spermatogenesis Formation of the sperm in the testes, by meiotic division of spermatozoa.

Spermatozoon A mature sperm cell.

Spermicide Substance that kills sperm and is used as a contraceptive method.

Spontaneous abortion Miscarriage; unintentional termination of pregnancy before the twentieth week.

Sterilization Permanent prevention of pregnancy.

Stricture Narrowing of a tubular structure, as an urethral stricture.

T

Teratogen Agent or factor that causes defects in the developing embryo.

Testicle See Testis.

Testis (testes) One of two organs of the male reproductive system located in the scrotum, in which the sperm and testosterone are made.

Testosterone The major male sex hormone, made by the cells of Leydig in the testes.

Thirst center Cells in the hypothalamus that are activated when the extracellular fluid volume is reduced. The stimulated cells produce the sensation of thirst.

Torsion In the testis, twisting of the spermatic cord.

Toxic shock syndrome (TSS) Acute bacterial infection that usually affects menstruating women who use tampons.

Transurethral resection Insertion of a resectoscope into the urethra, to cut away and remove part of the prostate gland.

Trichomoniasis Vaginal infection with trichomonad parasites.

Trophoblast cells Cells on the outer wall of the blastocyst, which develop into parts of the placenta.

Tubal ligation Sterilization technique in which the uterine tubes are severed.

Tubular reabsorption When water and solutes are returned to the blood stream during the process of urine formation.

Tubular secretion Movement of substances in the bloodstream from the peritubular capillaries into the tubules, to be excreted in the urine.

U

Umbilical cord Flexible structure that connects the embryo or fetus to the placenta.

Upper urinary tract infection Infection affecting the kidneys.

Ureter A tube 25 to 30 cm. long that carries urine from the kidney to the bladder.

Urethra Passage for urine from the bladder to outside the body.

Urethral stricture Narrowing of the urethra.

Urethritis Urethral inflammation, caused by highly acid urine, the presence of bacteria, or constriction of the urethral passage.

Urge incontinence Sudden uncontrollable urge to urinate.

Urinalysis Basic laboratory examination of the urine, including testing for urine concnetration, observation of color and clarity, basic chemical testing, and microscopic examination.

Urinary meatus Opening from the urethra to outside the body.

Urinary tract The kidneys, ureters, bladder, and urethra.

Urine creatinine test See creatinine clearance test.

Urine culture Incubation of a clean-catch-midstream urine specimen and counting and identification of any bacteria that grow.

Urologist Physician who deals with problems of male and female, child and adult urinary tracts, and with the male reproductive system.

Uterine prolapse Collapse of the uterus into the vagina.

Uterine tube or Fallopian tube One of two ducts through which ova travel from the ovary to the uterus.

Uterus Pear-shaped organ that holds and nourishes a developing fetus during pregnancy.

V

Vagina Canal that extends from the vulva to the cervix and receives the penis during intercourse.

Vaginitis Inflammation of the vagina.

Varicocele Swelling around the testis caused by constriction of the veins that carry blood away from the testis.

Vas deferens One of a pair of tubes leading from the epididymis to the ejaculatory duct of the seminal vesicle.

Vascular renal failure Kidney failure caused by interruption of blood flow to the kidney, caused by embolism, aneurysm, or severe hypertension.

Vasectomy Sterilization technique in which the vas deferens is cut or cauterized.

Vestibule Portion of the external female genitalia that lies inside the labia.

Vesicular ovarian follicle See Graafian follicle.

Vulva External female genitals, which include the labia majora, labia minora, and clitoris.

Vulvectomy Removal of a vulvar growth and surrounding tissue.

Vulvitis Inflammation of the vulva.

W

Wilms' tumor Kidney tumor (embryonal carcinosarcoma) usually affecting young children.

Y

Yolk sac Placental membrane that connects to the mother.

Z

Zona pellucida Tough membrane surrounding the ovum.

Zygote Cell resulting from the union of a sperm and an ovum.

papanicolaou (pap) smear
  defined, 134
papilla, 6
  defined, 134
parathormone, 14
parathormone defined, 134
parathyroid hormone, 14
  defined, 135
paraurethral, 73
paraurethral glands defined, 135
parity, 115
partial mastectomy, 90
parturition, 100, 110
  defined, 135
parturition disorders, 114–121
passive transport
  defined, 135
  term review, 11
pediatricians, 66
pelvic examination, 93
pelvic girdle, 68
pelvic inflammatory disease
  (PID), 83, 84, 86
  defined, 135
pelvis, 68, 69
penile wart, 51
  defined, 135
penis, 43
  cancer, 59
  defined, 135
percutaneous nephroscopy, 29
perineum, 73
peristalsis, 9
  defined, 135
peritoneal dialysis, 23
peritoneum, 4, 70
  defined, 135
peritonitis, 89
  defined, 135
peritubular capillary, 8
  defined, 135
pessary, 87, 88
  defined, 135
Peyronie's disease, 62
  defined, 135
pH balance, 14, 15
pH scale, 15
pheremones, 72
phimosis, 62
  defined, 135
PID (pelvic inflammatory disease), 83, 84, 86
PIH (pregnancy induced hypertension), 117
placenta, 103, 105, 106
  defined, 135
  formation, 104, 105
  previa, 116, 117
  previa defined, 135

placental stage, 112
placental vessels, 105
PMS (premenstrual syndrome), 83
pneumonocytis pneumonia, 55
polycystic kidney disease, 29, 30
polyuria, 24
  defined, 135
postpartal
  period, 112, 113
  psychological changes, 113
postrate gland, 42
postrenal failure, 32
  defined, 135
poststreptococcal disease, 25, 26
poststreptococcal glomerulonephritis defined, 135
potassium balance, 14
preeclampsia, 117
pregnancy, 68, 100
  date estimation, 100
  defined, 135
  diagnosis, 100, 101
  disorders, 114–121, 115
  ectopic, 115
  effects on mother, 109
  high blood pressure, 109
pregnancy-induced hypertension
  (PIH), 117
  defined, 135
premature delivery, 100
premature infant, 107
premature labor, 119–121
  defined, 135
premenstrual syndrome (PMS), 83
  defined, 135
prenatal care, 109, 110
prepuce, 44, 72
prerenal failure, 32
  defined, 135
pressure gradient term review, 11
priapism, 62
  defined, 135
progestrone, 69, 75
  defined, 135
prolactin, 113
  defined, 135
prolapsed umbilical cord, 119
prostate gland defined, 135
prostatectomy, 50
prostatic portion ejaculatory tube,
  43
prostatic portion of the urethra
  defined, 135
prostatic specific antigen (PSA),
  57
prostatitis, 50
  defined, 135
prostrate, 56, 57
  cancer, 57, 58

proximal convoluted tubule, 11
proximal tubule, 6, 11, 12
  defined, 135
PSA (prostatic specific antigen), 57
pubic lice, 56
pudendal, 121
pyelonephritis, 24
  defined, 135
pyramid, 6
  defined, 135
pyuria defined, 135

rapid plasma reagin (RPR) test, 53
reabsorption tubular, 11
rectocele, 88
  defined, 135
reflux defined, 135
renal artery, 5, 7
  defined, 135
renal calculus, 28, 29
  defined, 135
renal colic, 28
  defined, 135
renal column, 6
  defined, 135
renal corpuscle
  defined, 135
renal pelvis, 6
  defined, 135
renal threshold, 11
  defined, 135
renal vein, 5
  defined, 135
renin defined, 135
reproductive organs
  external, 69
  female internal, 69–72
  male, 40
reproductive structures, 40
resectoscope, 49
  defined, 135
resorption, 10
respiratory adjustments, 15
retroversion, 87
  defined, 135
rhythm method, 125
  defined, 135
RPR (rapid plasma reagin) test, 53
rugae, 9
  defined, 136

salpingitis, 85
  defined, 136
scrotum, 40
  defined, 136
second trimester, 106
secretion, 12
secundigravida, 115
semen, 42
  defined, 136

vulvectomy, 91
  defined, 137
vulvitis, 86
  defined, 137

water
  balance, 13

location in body, 13
  reabsorption, 11, 12
Western blot assay, 55
Wilms' tumor, 30
  defined, 137
withdrawal contraceptive
  method, 125

yolk sac, 103
  defined, 137

zidovudine (AZT), 55
zona pellucida, 102
  defined, 137
zygote, 102
  defined, 137